# strength training for runners

## avoid injury and boost performance

# strength training for
# runners

### avoid injury and boost performance

## John Shepherd

BLOOMSBURY
LONDON · NEW DELHI · NEW YORK · SYDNEY

Published by Bloomsbury Publishing Plc
50 Bedford Square
London WC1B 3DP
www.bloomsbury.com

ISBN (print): 978 1 4081 5561 5
ISBN (e-pdf): 978 1 4081 8142 3
ISBN (e-pub): 978 1 4081 8143 0

A CIP catalogue record for this book is available from the British Library.

**Acknowledgements**
Cover photograph © Getty Images
All inside images courtesy of Grant Pritchard with the exception of the following: pp. vi, 9, 62, 68, 79, 86, 171, 178 and 182–183 © Shutterstock images; p. 130 © istock image database; pp. 21, 27, 28, 29, 30 (bottom) 31, 32, 33, 34, 35 (top), 39, 40, 41, 42, 43, 75 and 149 © ultra-FIT magazine; pp. 18, 21 24, 35 (bottom), 36, 44, 48, 51–57, 61, 67 and 85, author's own
Illustrations by Tom Croft

Designed by James Watson
Commissioned by Charlotte Croft
Edited by Sarah Cole

This book is produced using paper that is made from wood grown in managed, sustainable forests. It is natural, renewable and recyclable. The logging and manufacturing processes conform to the environmental regulations of the country of origin.

Powerbag, ViPR, BOSU and Suspension Training are all registered trademarks

Typeset in MetaPlus by seagulls.net

Printed and bound in China by C&C Offset Printing Co

10 9 8 7 6 5 4 3 2 1

# contents

## acknowledgements

I would like to thank all those who have contributed to this project including the Bloomsbury editors, Sarah and Charlotte, the athletes in my training group, in particular Lauren Blackie who modelled for many of the photos, Premier Training whose facility we used for the gym-based shots, Steve Harrison who modelled and Grant Pritchard who took the photos in this location. Finally, very special thanks must go to Linda – my partner, who although not originally a runner, is now and has supported me throughout.

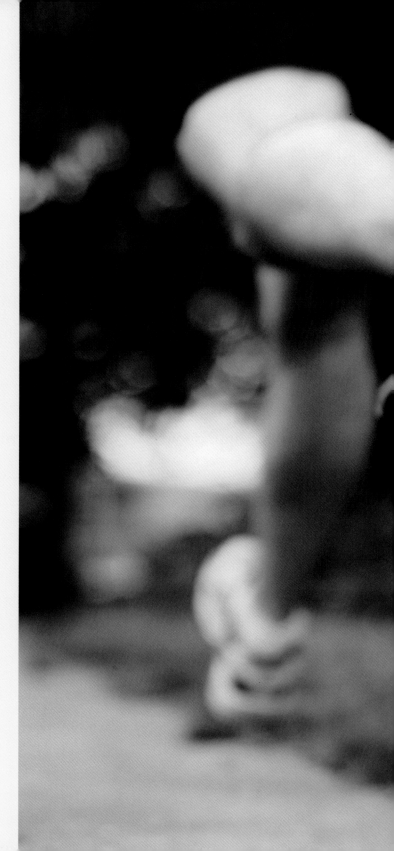

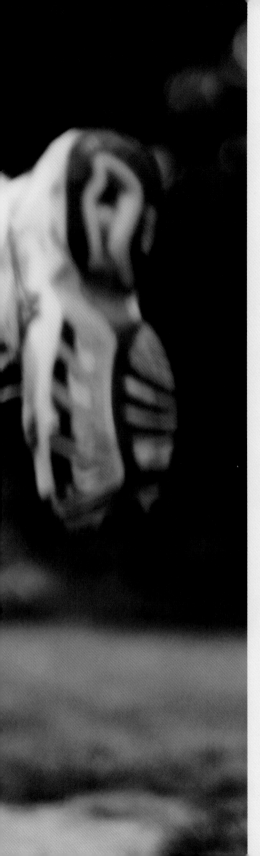

# introduction

Strength training is often ignored by the running fraternity, whose enjoyment largely derives from the activity itself and not from pumping iron or performing "fancy" sprint type drills on the track. However, when injuries occur enjoyment is certainly lacking and the longing to return to running can lead to negative feelings and even depression. However, with the "right" strength training approach in place – one that is balanced and reflects the needs and training and racing status of the runner – injury risk can be significantly reduced, with the added bonus that performance is also increased.

*Strength Training for Runners* is designed to keep you – as a runner – on track, on the road and out in the countryside, whatever your level or age. The chapters will guide you through the construction of a pre-conditioning routine that will iron out common running injuries, show you how to improve and strengthen your running (and other) muscles in your warm-ups, and provide you with some great conditioning advice that will make you a stronger and faster runner. The content of these later chapters focuses on circuit training, weight training, and plyometric training, for example. They include numerous examples of exercises and training programmes that are easy to follow and will improve your running and keep you off the physio's couch. Advice is also provided on how to construct a running-specific training programme, how to cross-train effectively and how to specifically train your core muscles.

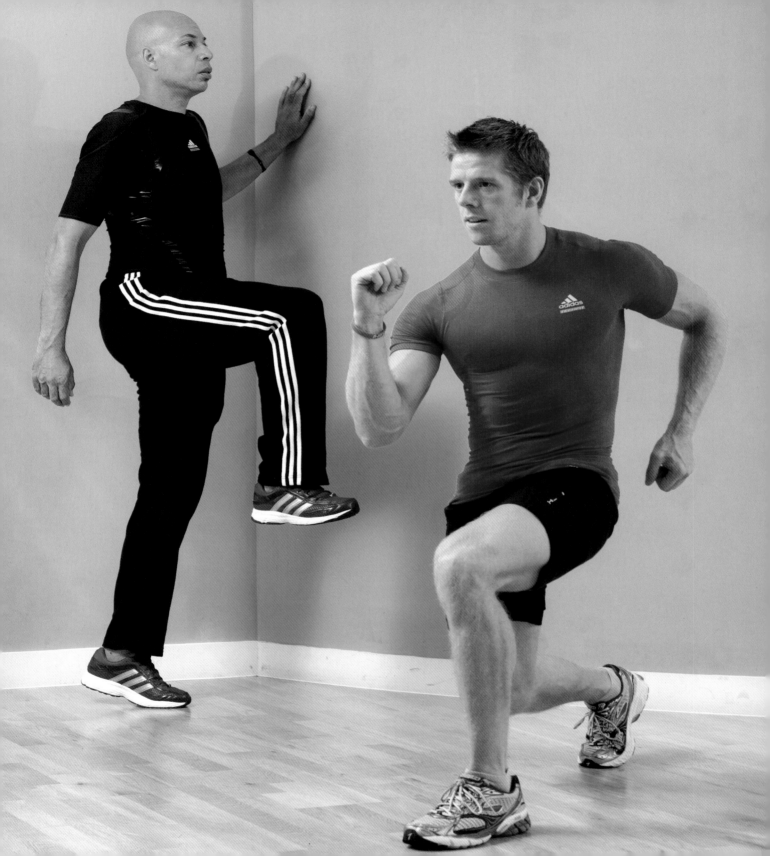

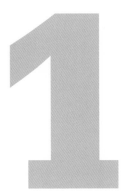

# pre-conditioning
## how to minimise your risk of running injury

## Laying the foundations

As a runner you'll probably be all too aware of the threat of injury. Very few of us who have been running for a number of years will have escaped without some form of ache, pain or something more serious. Running tends to create overuse injuries, which usually manifest themselves in the lower limbs and back area. More specifically, they can include "runner's knee", shin-splints, Achilles tendon problems, hamstring strains and heel pain (plantar fasciitis). Although these and other injuries often result from factors beyond the scope of this book, such as running in worn or the wrong (for your gait) trainers, too great an increase in training volume, changes to regular running surface or poor biomechanics (or any combination of the above), the good news is that you can do a great deal in your training to reduce their risk and keep them at bay.

Pre-conditioning (or pre-training) is a relatively new "buzz" word in the world of sports training. It refers to the process of "training to train" rather than training to compete or very directly improve performance. To help understanding, consider this: it's a bit like the preparatory processes followed in many manufacturing industries, where tolerances and tests are painstakingly devised for materials and structures, so that when they are finally incorporated into the end-product, the risks of failure are virtually nonexistent. In a not too dissimilar way, pre-conditioning techniques will extend the tolerances of your body and make it more robust to withstand potential running injuries.

## Implementing a running-specific pre-conditioning routine

Although GPs are becoming more enlightened, the chances are that if you were to go to one with a running injury, he/she would probably prescribe rest, physiotherapy, drugs and ultimately, should the injury not heal, surgery. However, unless you have a traumatic injury, many conditions can actually be "pre-conditioned away", or avoided in the first place. I'm not saying that the advice of the medical profession should be ignored – of course not, rather that you can take ownership of your own running health. Prevention in the case of running injuries, is very much better than cure.

Unless you are very unlucky and fall and break a bone or sprain an ankle, for example, the cause of most other running injuries is likely to be an intrinsic one. This is likely to result from your body type, sex and genetics, your running shoes and training environment (do you run on the roads or parkland most of the time?) and how you run (your gait). Pre-conditioning techniques can deal with the majority of these intrinsic factors.

Pre-conditioning for running involves self-testing, gait analysis and a repertoire of relevant strengthening exercises, and the start of the training year would seem an ideal time to pre-condition. Indeed, many running coaches would say that's what they are already doing by emphasising general training methods to build a foundation of strength for more specific work. In many ways these coaches are engaged in pre-conditioning, but in others they are not. Pre-conditioning should be implemented on an ongoing basis – it should operate continuously in the background of your main running programme in order to keep you in prime running condition all-year round. For example, bouts of eccentric calf training to "protect" against Achilles strain should be used periodically throughout the training year to keep this potential injury at bay (see table 1.2, page 7). A great time to implement this and other pre-conditioning exercises is during your warm-ups.

### How to pre-condition
#### *Understand your gait and your biomechanics*
Analysis of your running style can be a great eye-opener when it comes to tracing running-related injury problems and risk. Today, foot scans are relatively common in specialist running stores – their results will be interpreted to provide you with the best type of running shoes for your style of running and notably your foot strike. Slightly less prevalent are running biomechanics and conditioning experts who analyse your running action under very specific scrutiny. Invariably this will involve running on a treadmill while being filmed. It's an odd fact that many runners spend a great deal of time pondering over and designing their training plans, yet don't apply the same rigour to the

---

## Muscular actions

- A concentric muscular action occurs when a muscle shortens under load, for example, the biceps during the lifting part of a biceps curl.
- An eccentric muscular action occurs when a muscle lengthens under load, for example, the biceps during the lowering phase of the biceps curl.
- An isotonic muscular action involves movement and therefore concentric and eccentric muscular actions
- An isometric muscular action produces force but no movement

---

way they run. It's taken for granted that they "know" how to run. Often analysis throws up run technique idiosyncrasies, such as a splayed foot, tilted pelvis, shoulder rotation and so on, which can then be traced to previous aches, pains and injuries (or to likely causal factors for future ones). It's recommended that you seek the advice of running biomechanics experts and have your running style properly appraised as part of your pre-conditioning. A search on the internet will throw up a number of possibilities. See Chapter 2 for more information on running technique.

#### *Understand the muscular actions involved in running*
Understanding how your muscles work when running is very important. Running relies on a combination of moving (isotonic) concentric and eccentric muscular actions and also less obviously on held, isometric action (these occur when muscles work against each other, creating great tensions but no movement).

Eccentric muscle training can reduce the potential for Achilles tendon and hamstring injuries, for example. Eccentric contractions create more short- and long-term muscular damage than the concentric variety. Many runners will be all-too-familiar, for example, with

# Avoiding hamstring injury

In terms of learning from previous injuries, a team of researchers investigated hamstring injuries in elite athletes, hypothesising that those with a prior history of hamstring muscle strain were at increased risk of sustaining similar injuries in the future.[1] The research involved nine athletes with a history of hamstring injury and 18 uninjured athletes. Using specialised equipment, the researchers compared the torque that the hamstring muscles were subject to. Torque is force that creates twisting which, when it acts upon a muscle, can increase the risk of strain. The researchers discovered that torque peaked at much shorter muscle lengths in the injured athletes and recommended that in order to condition them against further injury, a combined programme of muscle testing and eccentric exercises should be implemented.

Not many coaches and runners have access to specialised equipment such as the isokinetic machinery required to test muscular strength used by the researchers, however, this should not be seen as a huge impediment to successful running pre-conditioning (and injury prevention), as you can implement some practical everyday methods available. Examples of eccentric strengthening drills for the hamstrings are provided on pages 31–2.

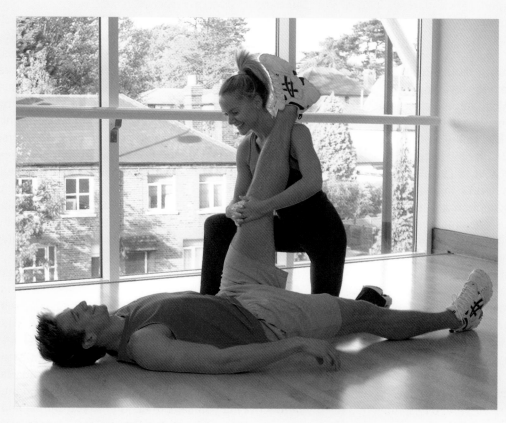

**Stretch to boost recovery and reduce injury**

the delayed onset of muscle soreness (DOMS) that occurs in the quadriceps (muscles to the front of the thighs) after downhill running. This results from the thigh muscles having to stretch on foot strike to control the speed of the descent (this is the eccentric load). It's possible to train your muscles to be better able to control eccentric forces – see pages 124 and 125.

### Understand why you get injured

Although the key to pre-conditioning is reducing injury risk, if you do sustain an injury it is important to understand why and take remedial steps to avoid a recurrence – this goal will form a significant part of future pre-conditioning programmes. In this respect, self-reflection and self-diagnostic tests can be used throughout your training to predict potential injury (see table 1.1, for an example of the latter), as can having a gait analysis under the watchful eye of an expert.

## Everyday pre-conditioning running tests
### Establish running strength and power levels

You can do this by testing, for example, for one-repetition weight training maximums (your one repetition maximum, or 1RM, refers to the maximum amount of weight you could lift only once on a specific exercise (see page 93 for how to calculate your own 1RM). Note that it is also possible to test for other set number maximums, for example 6 and 8). Doing this can provide a very useful pre-conditioning point of reference during your running conditioning as well. For example, if you have a large discrepancy in strength between your left and right legs and/or specific muscle groups, for example, hamstrings and quadriceps (the muscles of the back and front of the thigh respectively), then you could instigate a training programme designed to promote greater balance.

As will be indicated in subsequent chapters, performing strength training exercises will also increase your power output and enhance performance, while reducing injury potential.

### Use plyometric exercises

As with testing for disparities in strength levels using weights, you can also use plyometric (jumping) type exercises to achieve a similar purpose. For example, you could test how far you can hop on your left and your right leg and note the difference.

### Develop a repertoire of relevant pre-conditioning exercises – and know when to use them

Weight training as a pre-conditioner is covered later in this chapter and in more detail in chapter 8, while selected examples of pre-conditioning exercises are offered in table 1.2. Many of the drills identified in chapter 3 are also great pre-conditioners.

### Establish "norms" for your running-specific range of movement (ROM), i.e. specific flexibility

Injury is likely in key muscle and tendon groups, such as the hamstrings and Achilles tendons, if your specific flexibility is limited (although, as we will see, too much flexibility around joints can also be a problem – see page 49). This process will be subjective to some extent, particularly for novice runners with no training history, however, determining where muscular tightness could at best impair performance and at worst cause injury is key to successful pre-conditioning. Key muscle groups in this respect include the hamstrings, quads, calf muscles and hip muscles. Tight leg and hip muscles can lead to "runner's knee", for example, while hamstrings that are unable to stretch optimally eccentrically are more prone to injury – see page 3 for more detail.

### Analyse your running technique

Running appears to be a very simple activity – one that requires little skill. However, the more effective your running action is the better runner you will be and you'll also be less injury prone. In recent years there has been a big growth in gait analysis and biomechanical correction. Many sports shops offer foot scanners or similar devices designed to inform you about your running style and the way your foot contacts the ground. The aim is often to provide you with the best possible shoe choice. However, from a pre-conditioning standpoint the emphasis should be on looking for muscular imbalances rather than focusing on ways to enhance performance (although this is obviously also important and a derivative of relevant analysis).

Here's an example: when analysing a runner on a treadmill the focus could be on all of the following – hip alignment; the recovery phase of the running action (when the foot travels up towards your bottom, before being pulled through to the front); foot strike; and head, back and shoulder position – from study of the film it may be possible to discern such problems as a tilted pelvis, poor hamstring and hip flexor muscle strength (identified by a "lazier" lower leg return phase) or angled pelvis. You and/or your running coach can then design a training programme, using relevant pre-conditioning exercises to counteract this technical problem.

### Self-tests

Self-testing can be used to identify the potential onset of an injury. Numerous self-diagnostic trigger point (TP) tests are available to coaches and runners, although these should not be regarded as substitutes for proper sports medicine/physiotherapy interventions. TPs can flag up potential "problems" before they become acute, allowing the coach/runner to attempt to condition them out and/or seek appropriate professional help. Table 1.1 gives an example of a self-test for knee injury.

### Use eccentric training

Eccentric muscular damage is a long-term probability for a distance runner, especially when you enter your middle and latter years. Gradually your muscles' ability to stretch and recoil diminishes due to the accumulation of thousands and thousands of miles in your legs (or more specifically your muscles). It has been argued that this becomes particularly manifest in runs over 10 miles. Strengthening muscles to withstand eccentric damage through appropriate pre-conditioning (see below) can help reduce eccentric muscle damage and strains as can cross-training (see chapter 10).

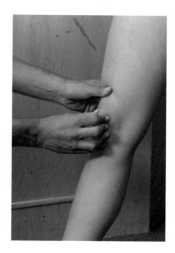

**How to test for "runner's knee"**

| Table 1.1 Trigger point self-diagnostic test to identify potential "runner's knee" | | |
|---|---|---|
| **Injury** | **Self-test** | **Method** |
| Patellofemoral pain syndrome (PFPS, or "runner's knee") | Palpating the knee cap | The coach uses his top hand to push down on the knee cap, lifting the lower pole of the patella. The thumb and forefinger of the lower hand then apply pressure to the lower borders of the inferior poles (sides) of the patella. If there is pain, it is more than likely that the |
| (See table 1.2 for a potential "treatment") | | athlete is suffering from/developing PFPS. |

*Adapted from Noakes (The Lore Of Running, 4th edition)*

**Examples of pre-conditioning exercises:**

1 Controlled bouts of downhill running to induce minimum muscular soreness. For example, 4–6 x 100m at 70 per cent effort with walk-back recovery.

2 Eccentric pre-conditioning drills. Drop and hold jumps performed from a sturdy platform around 70cm high. The emphasis of these jumps is just on the "landing and hold". Your muscles at the hips, knees and ankles will stretch eccentrically on impact.

3 Eccentric weight training, where the emphasis is placed on just the lowering phase of an exercise. For example, controlling the weight as it is lowered during a squat for a 5–10-second count.

*Use weight training*

Although as a runner you may not be a regular weight trainer, it is important for pre-conditioning purposes to include weight training (and other resistance exercises) in your training. This is because it can reduce the incidence of injury by strengthening soft tissue (muscles, ligaments and tendons). It is important to select the "right" exercises and follow an appropriate training programme – see subsequent chapter (and chapters 6, 7, 8 and 9) for specific exercises and routines.

Table 1.2 lists a selection of weight training, resistance and drill-type exercises that are great running pre-conditioners.

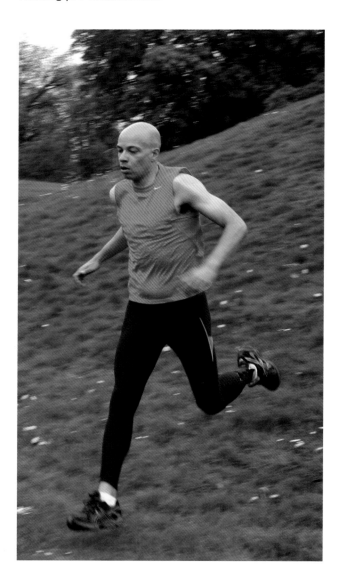

> ### ITB syndrome/'runner's knee' – further pre-conditioning suggestions
>
> 'Runner's knee' is often the result of a tight illiotibial band. This band of soft tissue runs along the outside of the thigh and can become tight, pulling on the ligaments that surround the knee. Simply applying a massage stick/roller to the outer portion of the thigh can flag up whether there is any soreness. The more acute this is the greater the potential for "runner's knee". Regular use of massage (using a massage stick/roller or via a sports masseuse) is a great pre-conditioning technique that can reduce the potential for this condition to develop (see pages 45 and 52 for selected examples).

**Table 1.2** Weight training and resistance exercises for running pre-conditioning

| Exercise | Preconditioning relevance | Comments/exercise pointers |
|---|---|---|
| Leg extension | Stabilises and strengthens the knee joint | Suitable for independent left and right leg training for more balanced strength development |
| Backwards and sideways running | Improves agility, lower limb strength, flexibility and kinesthetic awareness (the awareness of the body in space) | Can be included as a regular element of a warm-up |
| Eccentric calf raises | Strengthens Achilles tendons | (See panel on following page) |
| Dynamic standing leg cycling | Develops specific eccentric hamstring strength without the impact forces associated with running | Stand tall and cycle one leg underneath the body in an out-and-back running action. Use a wall to aid balance. Increase speed as confidence develops. The motion of the foot extending in front of the body and its arrest by the hamstrings is the prime cause of a hamstring strain (the eccentric contraction). This exercise pre-conditions against this. |
| Eccentric squats | Develops the absorbent strength of the thigh muscles and reduces injury risk | Set up a Smith machine so that it allows the weight to be lowered under control if using a heavy weight. You can perform the exercise with a lighter weight or even body weight. Lower to a 5-second count. |
| Single leg squat | Reduces the risk of "runner's knee" and improves balance | Stand on one leg and tuck the heel of the other up towards your bottom. Keeping your knee above your ankle and torso upright, squat down. Keep the heel firmly on the floor and push back up through it. Extend your hips at the top of the movement. Complete reps and perform on other foot. |
| Leg press | Reduces the risk of "runner's knee" | Seek expert advice if exercise causes pain |
| Ankle dorsi-flexion | Reduces potential for shin-splints | Sit and place an ankle weight around one foot. Keeping your heel on the ground, pull your toes up to your shins, hold and lower. Complete reps and perform on other foot. |

# Combat achilles tendon strain
## Why heavy weight training can make you a better runner

To further illustrate the role of weight training in pre-conditioning, let's consider the use of heavy load weight eccentric calf raises as a means of combating Achilles tendon injury. Many regular runners suffer from Achilles tendon problems at some stage in their running lives.

Tendinosis is the technical term used to describe the degeneration of Achilles tendon tissue, while Achilles tendinitis refers to inflammation of the soft tissue. Most Achilles pain is now believed to be a consequence of the former, particularly in runners who have numerous years of training behind them. Research found that heavy weight eccentric calf lowering exercises were a great treatment in research on two matched groups of 15 recreational athletes, both suffering from long-term Achilles tendinosis.[2]

The first group performed the heavy calf lowering exercises with an emphasis on the eccentric (lowering) phase, while the other received 'normal' physiotherapy treatment. At the end of the 12-week training programme, the weight-training group was able to run at pre-injury levels. By contrast, the group who did not perform the calf lowering exercises did not respond to physiotherapy and ultimately needed surgical treatment.

By now you will have become aware that training to train by way of following a pre-conditioning routine is highly important. You need to have a full understanding of running from a biomechanical and physiological basis in order to beat injury. This knowledge should lead to the development of a relevant pre-conditioning regime.

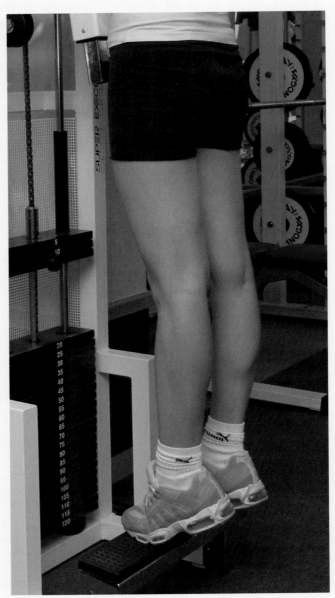

**Emphasising the lowering phase can reduce Achilles injury**

## Gender differences

Male and female runners can suffer from different types of injury and this makes for a further pre-conditioning consideration. For example, female athletes have a 4–7 times greater risk of developing an anterior cruciate ligament (ACL) injury than their male counterparts playing at similar levels in the same sports. This is because of female-specific differences in hip and lower limb alignment, which can lead to increased twisting forces being absorbed through the knee in women. The ACL is one of the four main knee ligaments and is often damaged by twisting and turning movement.

A great deal of research has been carried out into this vital area for pre-conditioning, which has resulted in a plyometric training programme being devised to reduce the incidence of knee damage in female athletes.[3] Females are much less able to withstand eccentric loading when jumping compared to males and therefore need more technical attention. Teaching proper biomechanics and following a specific strengthening routine involving, for example, eccentric exercises and paying particular attention to hamstring strength was found to significantly reduce the incidence of ACL injury in women.

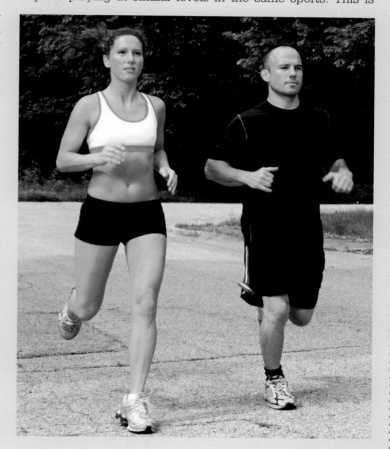

**Males and females can suffer from different types of running injury**

## References

1   *Medicine and Science in Sports and Exercise*, 2004 Mar; 36(3):379-87
2   *American Journal of Sports Medicine*, 1998 May-Jun; 26(3):360-6
3   *American Journal of Sports Medicine*, 1996 Nov-Dec; 24(6):765-73

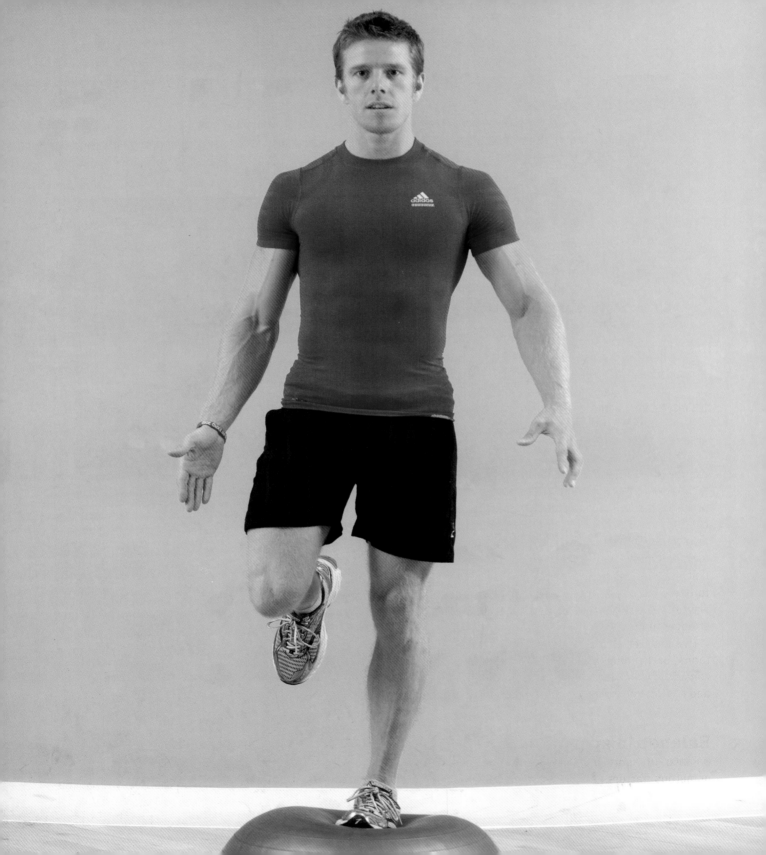

# 2

# balanced running
## how to run optimally

It's often said that the best runners are the best balanced – they seem to move with effortless grace, with each stride pushing them purposefully onward with little wasted effort. In chapter 3, you will find numerous examples of running drills that will improve your running technique and also specifically strengthen you in the process. However, it's important – particularly in the context of avoiding injury – to consider the mechanisms involved in balance and specialist exercises that can be used to improve your balance and running technique. In doing so you will gain a greater understanding of how to use specific balance exercises in your training in a way that will reduce injury potential and make you a stronger runner.

This chapter also considers the role of your feet in terms of keeping you running strong, including a consideration of the recent trend for barefoot running and minimalist shoes.

## Balance in sport

Balance in sport involves a complex interplay of numerous factors. Many are conscious – such as deciding to move a limb to prevent yourself falling – while many more are unconscious. When we run our body computes numerous calculations to keep us upright and in control of our running. This unconscious element involves the "use" of in-built sensory mechanisms and programmed responses. These are collectively known as "proprioception". Proprioception has been called the "sixth sense" – and is basically a mechanism (or more accurately series of mechanisms) that keeps track and control of muscle tensions and movement across our body and makes constant adjustments.

When we consciously make movements or are subjected to external forces, our muscles, ligaments and joints make their own "judgments" based on the information they receive from their own sources (receptors) as well as those we "ask" them to make, i.e. moving one leg in front of the other to run (from our conscious brain). These judgments are then used to switch on mechanisms to control movement (of which more later). These are specifically known as "sensorimotor processes" and sports scientists have been investigating how the senses consciously and subconsciously react with one another to control movement (known as "sensorimotor research").

It is now believed that sensiromotor ability and proprioception can be enhanced by specific practices. If you as a runner improve your sensiromotor ability, then you will not only be less likely to fall in the worst case scenario, but you will have a "better balanced" body that will be that much more effective as a running machine. This could enhance your off-road running, for example, where underfoot conditions create instability, by reducing the chances of you turning an ankle.

## Mechanics of proprioception

As we have seen, proprioception is achieved through muscles, ligaments and joint actions using messages that are continuously sent through the central nervous system (CNS). The CNS then relays information to the rest of the body, literally "telling" it how to react and with what amount of tension/action. Some of these instructions go to the brain where more often than not they are acted on consciously, while others go to a "control centre" located in the spinal cord, where they are acted on automatically.

Proprioceptors are essentially "sensors" within muscles, joints and ligaments. These respond to pressure, stretch and tension, and are key to initiating what is known as the "stretch reflex". You'll probably be familiar with the stretch reflex as a mechanism when trying to stretch a limb beyond its sticking point – a point will be reached when you'll not be able to stretch your leg, for example, any further. This is the result of the stretch reflex mechanism kicking in and putting a brake on your efforts to further stretch your muscle/muscles.

Although not as obvious, the stretch reflex also provides control over other functions in our body, for example, our postural muscles, which maintain the balance of the body against gravity. This makes the stretch-reflex a global muscle mechanism as well as a specific site one.

## Muscle spindles – the key to proprioception

Muscle spindles are the key to proprioception because they provide the information necessary for the CNS to produce the stretch reflex and attempt to ensure bodily control and stability.

Muscle spindles are special muscle fibres. There are more of them in muscles and muscle groups that perform complex movements, such as those for the hands and feet.

There are actually two types of fibre within muscle spindles. Intrafusal fibres are particularly crucial to proprioception as they have the ability to contract and adjust to the load the muscle is subject to in order to retain safe/effective posture. This is achieved by sending greater numbers of excitatory impulses to the prime mover muscles that need to control the movement and less to those that do not (the antagonists). Crucial to this process is a specific motor neuron in the spinal cord. This is called the efferent motor neuron. It is similar to the engine management system in a modern car because it controls all the information it receives and literally adjusts the power output of the body's muscles to maintain safety and integrity.

Ligaments also contain proprioception mechanisms called the Golgi tendon organs. These also have the ability to monitor muscular tension and they also send messages to the spinal cord, which are then returned in an attempt to put the "brakes" on a muscle group being overstretched. This is achieved by sending out inhibiting electrical signals to the muscle.

Here's an example: if you were holding a weight in your outstretched hand and then you suddenly added more load, the stretch reflex would attempt to make the adjustments necessary to allow you to continue to hold the added load by "tweaking" all the supporting muscles and influencing your posture.

## Injury can impair proprioception

Injury can reduce the effectiveness of your proprioception abilities – this is something that you may not be fully aware of, even when your rehabilitation seems complete and you're back to your running. Researchers looked at the role of the sensiromotor system and its relation to functional stability, joint injury and muscle fatigue of the shoulder and the restoration of functional stability after shoulder injury.[1] They noted that to fully restore shoulder stability, deficits in mechanical stability, proprioception and neuromuscular control were needed. Examples of training methods for restoring and enhancing proprioception for the lower leg – a site that runners commonly injure – can be found in table 2.1.

### Slow and fast twitch muscle fibre, proprioception and balance drills

Weight training (and other resistance training options) is crucial to runners for enhancing running speed and reducing injury. Maximum strength and power weight training help to develop fast twitch muscle fibres. These are our speed and power producing muscle fibres. Plyometric and sprint training also target fast twitch muscle fibre. However, too great an emphasis on the development of fast twitch muscle fibre can disrupt proprioceptive ability. This is because fast twitch muscle fibre is less adept at monitoring and controlling muscle tension than slow twitch (endurance type) fibre, because of the quicker speed of neural impulses being sent and interpreted through muscle spindles and spinal motor neurons by the former.

Performing more balance-oriented exercises at slower paces will enhance proprioception, as they will allow postural stabiliser muscles, which have a greater predominance of slow twitch muscle fibre, to help with movement control. It is therefore important that you include exercises that target all types of muscle fibre in your running resistance/pre-conditioning strengthening programme.

An example of a stabilising slow twitch fibre-rich muscle is the soleus muscle of the calf. The other major calf muscle, the larger gastrocnemius, is the fast twitch fibre-rich prime mover. It provides the power and the soleus the control.

Balance type drills not only help you to enhance proprioception and reduce potential injury, but they can paradoxically help to make you a faster, stronger runner. Next time you're running with a group of runners look, if you can (without tripping!), at the way their feet strike the ground and what the lateral, side-to-side movements as manifested in the hip/lower back region, shoulders, knees and hips in particular looks like. If you spot twisting movements around the ankles, knees and hips, then it's likely that balance mechanisms, specific strength and poor running technique are all contributory factors. The more effective your sensiromotor abilities and your stabilising muscles are, the more effective the power output will be from the prime movers, which all helps to make you a faster, stronger and more injury resilient runner.

### Back strength and proprioception development

Swiss balls are great training tools for developing greater proprioceptive ability and enhanced postural stability – they can be found in most gyms and are relatively inexpensive to purchase for home use. Back injuries and soreness are common among runners, so specific Swiss ball exercises and more specific core work (see chapter 9) will make for more robust running.

**Table 2.1** Progression of selected proprioception developing exercises for rehabilitation after injury and/or to improve ankle and lower leg strength and stability

| Exercise | Description | Comments |
|---|---|---|
| Standing double leg balance with eyes closed | Simply stand flat footed for 15 seconds or more with eyes closed | This simple exercise would be one of the first to be used when regaining/improving proprioception after an ankle injury. The lack of visual cues will enhance proprioception, as you have to stay on the spot. |
| Single leg balance from tiptoes | Tuck the heel of one foot up towards your bottom and extend onto the toes of the other foot, balance for 15 seconds | Performed from one leg and on tiptoes, the balance requirement is significant. There is likely to be more "sway" which will need to be controlled, firing greater numbers of proprioceptors. |
| Single leg balance with eyes closed, performed flat footed or on tiptoes | As above, but with eyes closed and from a flat foot stance | As with the first exercise, the lack of visual cues will require greater proprioception, as will the unilateral nature of the exercise |

| | | | |
|---|---|---|---|
| Standing double leg balance on wobble board/BOSU | 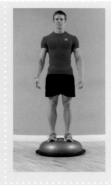 | Stand feet astride of the wobble board/BOSU and attempt to balance, hold for 15 seconds plus | Now, the "ground" becomes unstable and the wobble factor increases. Proprioceptors and stabilising muscles will have to work harder to retain balance. |
| Standing double leg balance on wobble board/BOSU with eyes closed | 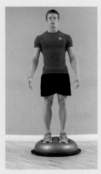 | Hold for 15 seconds | The lack of visual cues further enhance proprioception requirements |
| Single leg wobble board/BOSU balance | 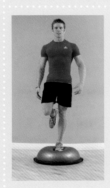 | Hold for 15 seconds plus | This progression obviously enhances the proprioceptive requirements of the exercise |
| Single leg stance on wobble board/BOSU while catching and throwing ball | 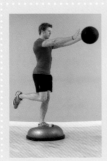 | 2 x 10 catches | The addition of the throw and catch unsettles balance even more and requires greater unconscious proprioception as focus is placed on the ball skill. The ball can be thrown using a chest pass action against a wall for the rebound to be caught or to a partner. Throws can be made from the chest and forwards or, for added difficulty, the ball can be thrown at arm's length from the side of the body. |

## Ex 2.1 Incline pelvic tilt to strengthen and stabilise the core

**Benefits**

This exercise strengthens your abdominals and back muscles and improves pelvic control and range of movement.

**How to perform**

Sit upright on the Swiss ball with knees bent and feet flat on the floor. Walk your feet out in front of you until you are lying with the ball in the middle of your back. Your hips should be off the ball and your feet shoulder-width apart. Lower your hips onto the ball. Keep your neck and shoulders relaxed. Using your abdominal muscles to initiate the movement, tilt your pelvis upward to lift your hips off the ball. Slowly bring your hips back down onto the ball, still using your abs and keeping your spine in a neutral (not overly rounded or arched) position.

*Do: 2 sets of 15 reps.*

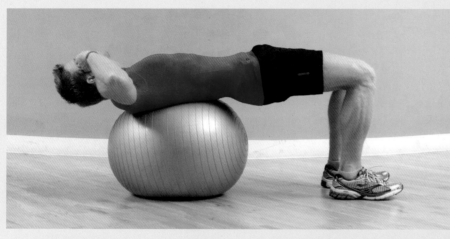

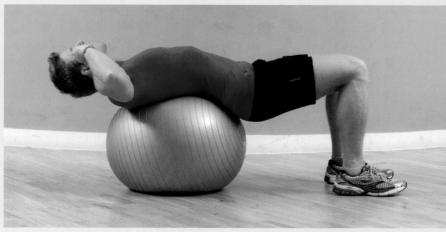

## Ex 2.2 Single leg balance, using Swiss ball while holding medicine ball

**Benefits**
This exercise strengthens the abdominal and back muscles.

**How to perform**
The goal of the exercise is to stabilise your back against the Swiss ball and turn against the wall. Hold the medicine ball at arm's length, which will also activate postural proprioceptors, while the supported leg has to "root" itself to the spot to hold the movement together.

**Progressions**
This exercise can be progressed by moving the medicine ball from side to side, by throwing and catching a ball from this position, or by performing a controlled single leg squat (see photo).

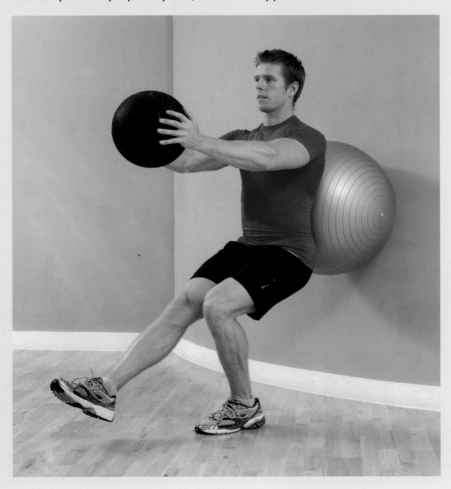

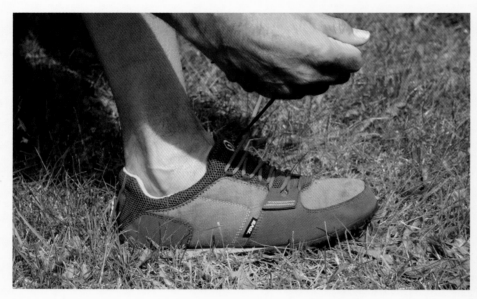

**Minimalist shoe**

# Barefoot/minimalist shoe running

Your feet are the foundations for your running and it stands to reason that the stronger they are the better your running will be.

Those of us of a certain age will recall plimsolls – those very flimsy shoes that had millimetres of cushioning and were flat, i.e. there was no rear foot, mid-sole nor forefoot cushioning. Yet tens of thousands of us ran in them and did all manner of sports – without injury. In a way they were minimalist shoes in an age when the concept had not even been born. Had we not been encouraged by shoe companies designing shoes which said that more cushioning is better, it's possible that we'd be running better, as nature intended and possibly with less running-related injury problems.

Recently there has been an explosion in barefoot running and shoes that are minimalist in design that provide little support in comparison to traditional running shoes. Some of these are designed to fit your feet like gloves and only provide protection from sharp objects, for example, when running, while others offer slightly more protection (they often come in "grades" of flexibility, cushioning and protection), so that you can become gradually accustomed to running with little support over a period of time, by moving through shoe grades.

### Forefoot running

The minimalist/barefoot approach goes hand in hand with an emphasis on forefoot running. Forefoot running, as its name suggests, results in foot-strikes being made on the front portion of the feet (with the heel making little or no contact with the ground). This creates greater momentum and allows the body to better cushion force using its own structures. Proponents believe that this produces faster running and less shock travels through the body. This is because the built-up, cushioned heel that traditional running shoes have simply doesn't get in the way as the foot strike takes place. When you are wearing running shoes, the tendency for most is to heel-strike, to literally "plonk" down into the heel. But doing this sends greater vertical forces through the body, increases ground contact time, reduces the foot's natural ability to dissipate force and is therefore less efficient in terms of generating speed.

### Feeling the ground

A very high proportion of running injuries result in injuries to the ankle, often caused by twisting/turning of the ankle. Normal running shoes can contribute to this by reducing the effectiveness of your proprioceptive abilities. As we have seen, they take away much of the "feel" that running in barefoot or minimalist shoes provides. Contemporary running shoes are also relatively unstable on unstable surfaces, such as parkland (obviously there are shoes that are designed for different conditions, such as fell running shoes, which are actually very unstructured), but overall the mid-sole in traditional running shoes acts in a way that can make stability, particularly on uneven surfaces, difficult. This is because your foot sits high above the ground on a wide cushion and is divorced from the running surface.

### Joining the barefoot/minimalist shoe movement

I am an advocate of incorporating aspects of the barefoot/minimalist shoe movement in your training in order to strengthen and improve balance, for example; however, this must be done slowly and progressively. One of the easiest and most low impact ways is to perform running drills barefoot or in socks or in minimalist shoes on a suitable surface, such as a running track or gymnasium floor. The best drills to start with are those that are relatively static and have reduced impact, such as walking lunges, marches and the walking running action (see chapter 3). After a period of time, jogging barefoot over very short distances as part of your warm-up could be introduced.

Barefoot or minimalist running shoe running will also improve proprioception and "teach" your body how to respond better to different underfoot conditions. It's also possible that the chances of sustaining the common running injury plantar faciitis (inflammation of the ligament running along the bottom of the foot) could be reduced.

However, I would steer clear of aiming to run your next marathon (or race of any distance) barefoot or relatively unshod. Our bodies have evolved to "want" to wear shoes and they do get some benefit from the cushioning provided. However, budget permitting, always be sure to get the right running shoes for your gait and for the type of running you do and strengthen your feet and other running muscles by careful use of minimalist shoes/barefoot drills.

## The merits of barefoot running

Although research into the merits of barefoot running versus shoe running is only just reaching a viable level for cross evaluation, it seems that barefoot running will reduce the forces the body is subject to.

Researchers from Harvard University discovered that "even on hard surfaces, barefoot runners who forefoot strike generate smaller collision forces than shod rearfoot strikers. This difference results primarily from a more plantar-flexed (toes down) foot at landing and more ankle compliance during impact, decreasing the effective mass of the body that collides with the ground … (barefoot or minimal running shoes) may protect the feet and lower limbs from some of the impact-related injuries now experienced by a high percentage of runners."[1]

## Lower leg and proprioception development

### Muscles of the lower leg

The main lower leg muscles are the larger gastrocnemius and the smaller soleus. Both contribute to ankle movement. The "gastroc" is the larger of the two and resides on the outer portion of the lower leg, when viewed from the back. The soleus is smaller and is positioned to the inside. The muscles interact with the ankle joint through a myriad of smaller muscles that stabilise and control the movement of this joint and the foot. Crucial in this respect is the Achilles tendon. This band of soft tissue connects the heel bone to the calf muscles. It acts as a kind of cable that "pulls" on the heel, through the action of the calf muscles, to create ankle movement. It also has crucial shock absorption and energy return roles, which can significantly contribute to the development of running power.

To the front of the lower legs, running over and around the shin, are further muscles such as the peroneus longus, and tendons such as the extensor hallucius longus.

The foot contains over 100 muscles ligaments and tendons and 24 bones.

### How the muscles of the lower leg contribute to walking, running and sprinting

There is considerable research to show how the muscles of the lower leg contribute to walking, running and sprinting. Let's look at the role of the main lower leg muscles involved in walking. Researchers examined the individual contributions of the gastrocnemius and soleus muscles at a walking speed of 1.5m/s. At any instant in the gait cycle (the walking or running action), the contribution of these muscles to supporting the body and moving it forwards was defined by their contribution to the trunk's vertical and horizontal velocity and its contribution to moving the legs forward during the swing phase of the gait cycle. Vertical velocity refers to the movement of the body upwards and downwards across the curvilinear path of the running stride. Horizontal momentum refers to the movement forwards across the running surface. Too much vertical input will slow the runner by creating a heavy-style and too much horizontal input will result in shortened strides. During the stance phase (when one foot is on the ground) the body is normally held in an upright position. Looking at the lower leg muscles the researchers found that the gastrocnemius and soleus provided trunk support during the single leg stance and pre-swing (the moment when the leg swings into the next stride) phases of the walking action. As the body moves into early single leg stance, the gastrocnemius and soleus accelerate the trunk vertically but decelerate forward progression of the trunk. In mid single-leg stance, the gastrocnemius delivers energy to the leg, while the soleus decelerates it, however their function is reversed for their action on

The gait cycle

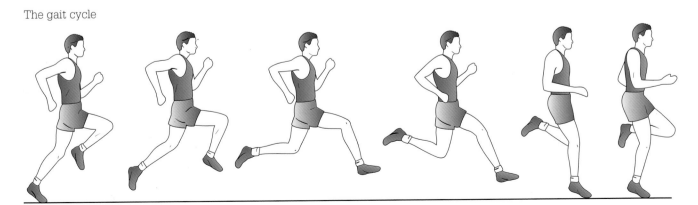

the trunk. In the late single leg stance, just prior to the foot leaving the ground, both major calf muscles perform a concentric muscular action as they accelerate the trunk forward while decelerating the downward motion of the trunk (basically they act to prevent the ankle collapsing back to the floor).

## Running and sprinting

The action of the lower leg muscles is very similar during running and sprinting compared to walking, although the hip muscles play a far greater role in generating speed in terms of the upper legs.[2] Sprinting, in particular, also involves far greater impact forces than walking (up to three time plus body weight), although the foot may only be in contact with the ground for 0.089 of a second for an elite sprinter. During the foot strike, pre- and mid-stance phases, the calf muscles have to absorb this force before contributing to pushing the athlete forward into the next stride, while stabilising their trunk (akin to walking, but as noted with a far greater shock absorbency and reactive requirement). The calf muscles work with the Achilles tendons to absorb and return this force. This is achieved by a lengthening eccentric muscular action. Sports scientists refer to "joint stiffness" when it comes to promoting greater speed – faster runners have greater joint stiffness – think of using a "pogo stick made of jelly" (!) rather than one made from very resilient rubber; the latter will of course return much more energy than the former.

Using another analogy, it is akin to throwing a golf ball against a wall – the harder the ball is thrown, the greater the speed of the ball returning from the wall will be, due to the elastic properties of the ball. However, if the ball were made of foam, no matter how hard the throw, the ball's return would be very weak. Your legs need to be resilient and elastic – possess greater stiffness (as the sports scientists say) – to optimise your running speed.

Sports scientists argue that during sprinting the prime role of the ankle (and knee) is to create high joint stiffness before and during the contact phase, while

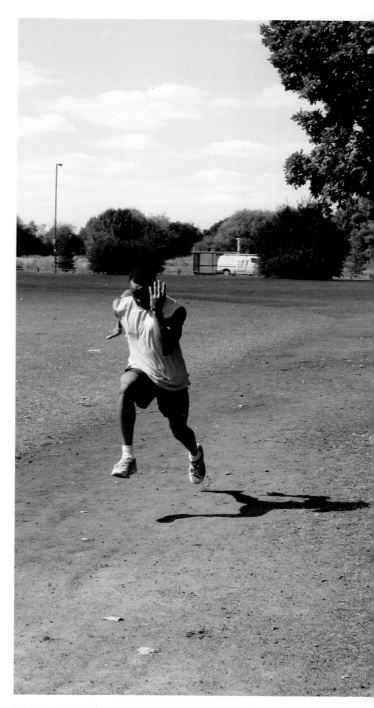

Sprinting and running obviously share similar dynamics

21

the hip flexors (muscles at the tops of the thighs) function as the prime forward movers of the body.[3]

Being too flexible around your joints was indicated as being a potential impediment to faster running in chapter 1 – the information on joint stiffness presented above helps to clarify why this is the case (sprinting as a way to enhance your running strength and performance is covered in chapter 6).

## Reducing injury through lower limb strengthening

There are lots of exercises that can be used to strengthen the lower limbs. Some of these are shown on pages 14 and 15.

Researchers looked at how ankle (and knee) injuries could be reduced in Norwegian teenage handball players during the 2002/2003 season.[4] The survey involved 1837 players, who were split into an intervention group (958 players) and a control group (879 players). The former performed exercises designed to improve awareness and control of the ankles and knees during standing, running, dynamic lateral movements, jumping and landing. The exercises included a warm-up, use of a ball and wobble boards, and focused on sport technique, balance and strength. Players spent 4–5 minutes on each group of exercises for a total of 15–20 minutes for the first 15 training sessions and thereafter once per week. Coaches recorded attendance and details of the sessions. The control group continued with their normal training methods. So what did the team discover?

During the season, 262 players (14 per cent) were injured at least once (241 acute and 57 overuse injuries). Of these the intervention group had lower risks than the control group when it came to sustaining acute knee or ankle injuries. The occurrence for moderate and major injuries (defined as absence from play for 8–21 days) were also lower for the intervention group for all injuries. Risk of injury did not differ between men and women.

The researchers concluded that, "The rate of acute knee and ankle injuries and all injuries to young

## Tendons produce running power

You may well assume that it's your legs, notably your thighs, which are the running muscles. Although they do supply considerable power, mainly through concentric muscular actions, tendons – and especially the Achilles tendons – are crucial in this respect (as are the hip flexor muscles). These structures store and return elastic energy into each and every step and are subject to the highest loads in the body when running and jumping.

Plyometric training can boost the power output of muscles and their supporting tendon structures (these jumping type exercises and their relevance to running are covered in greater detail in chapter 8). However, many runners stay away from these types of exercises as they believe that they will have little direct impact on running performance.

In the grand scheme of things an effective cardiovascular system with a high $VO_2$max and lactate threshold are the main determinants of endurance running performance (the former refers to the maximum amount of oxygen your body can process, measured either in litres per minute or in millilitres per minute per kilo of body weight) and the latter to the maximum pace you can sustain aerobically – when you exceed your lactate threshold, your body will supply a greater portion of its energy anaerobically. However, if the legs can be made more dynamic, then each and every stride will be longer and potentially quicker. In fact, research has found that the fastest 10k runners are often the fastest of their peers when racing over 40m.

handball players was reduced by half by a structured programme designed to improve knee and ankle control during play."

As a runner, the demands placed on your ankles and knees will not be the same as the handball players, but the take-home value is very similar in that it is very worthwhile performing relevant "protective" exercises.

### Even a toe can make a difference!

Feet (and toes) can influence running power and reduce injury potential. Researchers studied the energy contribution of the big toe (metatarsophalangeal (MP) joint) when running and sprinting.[5] They wanted to discover what the contribution of the MP joint was to the total mechanical energy involved in running and sprinting. Data was collected from 10 trained male athletes (5 runners and 5 sprinters). The team discovered that during the stance phase the joint absorbed large amounts of energy (on average 20.9 Joules during running and 47.8J during sprinting). In terms of biomechanics this led them to conclude that lack of plantar flexion (toe-down position) of the MP joint resulted in a lack of energy generation during take-off – energy was absorbed at the joint and dissipated in the shoe and foot structures and was not returned to propel the athlete forward. Although it is difficult to specifically train the big toe to contribute more to the sprint and running action, concentrating on a more dorsi-flexed foot-up position on foot strike could allow it (and the foot structure in general) to generate more propulsive force, as the firmer position would prime the lower leg muscles for greater force/energy return.

## Foot and toe strengthening exercises

## Toe clawing
### How to perform

Stand barefoot on a carpet. Scrunch the toes of one foot and try to claw/pull yourself forward. Persevere, as you will be able to achieve some forward

## Plyometric training and its effects on running times

Researchers looked specifically at plyometric training and its affects on 3k time. Seventeen runners were randomly placed into a group that did six weeks of plyometric training and one that did not. Both groups performed similar running training. It was discovered that the plyometric training runners' times over 3k were 2.6 per cent better than those who did no plyometrics. This improvement in running economy was attributed to the plyometric training as other variables, such as $VO_2max$ and lactate threshold, showed no variation between the groups of runners.[6]

movement in time. Once you have mastered this, continue to toe-pull yourself forward, using each foot in an alternate fashion (see also barefoot/minimalist shoe running, pages 18–19).

## Performing sprint drills and running barefoot/in minimalist shoes

As indicated, the feet can also be strengthened by performing sprint drills barefoot and even by running (although you should progress carefully to the latter).

## References

1   *Nature*, 2010 Jan 28; 463(7280):531-5
2   *Journal of Biomechanics*, 2001 Nov; 34(11):1387-98
3   *Journal of Sports Sciences*, 2001 Apr; 19(4):263-72
4   *Medicine and Science in Sports and Exercise*, 1981; 13(5):325-8
5   *Journal of Biomechanics*, 1997 Nov-Dec; 30(11-12): 1081-5
6   *European Journal of Applied Physiology*, 2003 Mar; 89(1):1-7; E Pub 2002 Dec 24

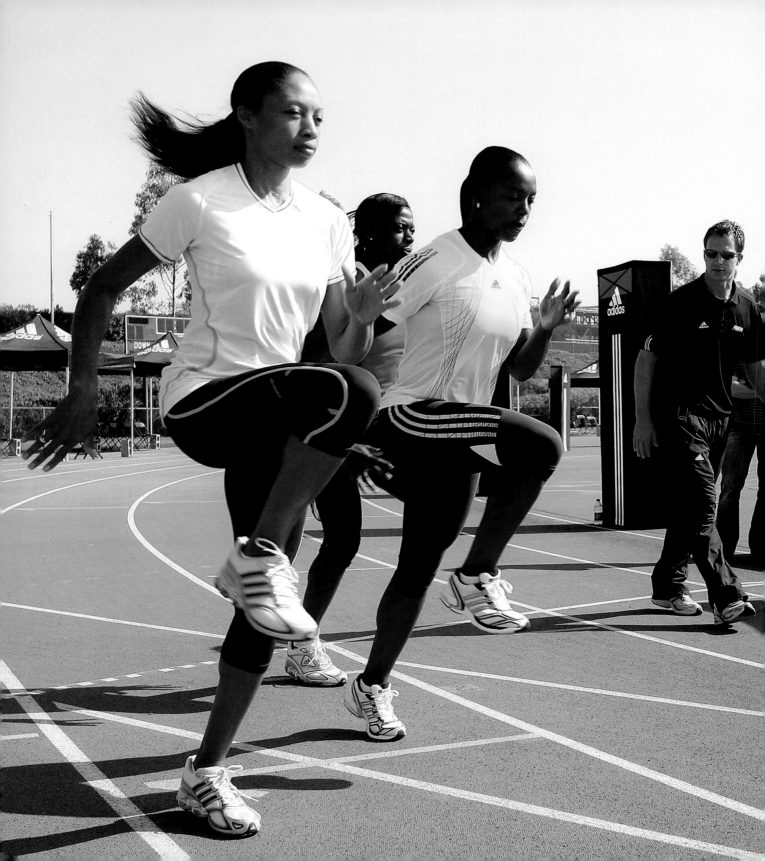

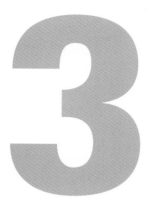

# running drills

improve your technique
and specific strength

Putting one foot in front of the other to run should be simple. But if it were, we'd all be super-fit runners striding purposefully around the streets and across the countryside powered by our endurance engine and benefiting from a silky smooth stride. A look at any mass participation running race will show that this is far from the case. Regularly performing running drills, coupled with specific resistance exercises, can improve your technique and strengthen key running muscles reducing injury potential (further relevant exercises are provided in chapter 4).

## The drills

The drills that follow target the various points in the running stride and should all help you perfect a good running style. These are:

- The foot-strike phase
- The recovery phase
- The drive phase

We also look at selected arm action drills to go alongside the running stride drills.

All drills should be performed on a suitable surface, such as a running track, dry flat grass or in a sports hall. They are designed to improve technique, therefore, it is best that they are performed with quality. Fatigue will impair the accuracy and precision of movement, so be sure to avoid getting tired by taking plenty of recovery. If fatigue sets in, then reduce your reps or the distance over which you perform the drills – if you don't, you could end up learning the "wrong" movement patterns.

Before performing the drills warm up with 5 minutes of jogging and then perform functional movements (i.e. movements that mimic how you will use the body in the drills) for all body parts, such as marching on the spot and arm swings. Cool down with a couple of minutes of jogging and stretch out your major body parts.

## Foot-strike phase drills

On foot-strike the foot normally rolls in to absorb impact forces – this is known as pronation. If the foot rolls in too far, this is known as over-pronation and injuries can result. It is therefore important to have your gait checked by a suitably qualified person. Many

# Key running technique tips

- Look straight ahead and keep your chin and chest elevated.
- Use your arms to assist your running, particularly when running above three quarter pace (at lower speeds, let them follow your legs as pumping them powerfully will expend energy unnecessarily).
- Avoid twisting movements in your trunk, although there has to be some rotation due to the one leg at a time unilateral nature of the running action, however, this should be kept to a minimum. Too much rotation results in a loss of propulsive force (as energy is absorbed and wasted in the core and not transferred directly to the running surface). A weak non-running conditioned core often manifests itself in "core twisting" while running (see chapter 8 for numerous exercises to strengthen your core).
- Knees should be driven forwards and up (not just up – taken in extremis this would result in you running on the spot!). Your hip flexor muscles (the

muscle at the top front of your thigh) are crucial in this respect.
- Drive through your hip to push yourself forward. However, do not over exaggerate this otherwise you will potentially lope along by over striding.
- Try to strike the ground with your feet under your hips (this is called the stance phase, when one foot is grounded and the other is swinging into the next stride).
- Try to strike the ground towards your forefeet rather than on your heels (as has been noted throughout this book, modern running shoes tend to encourage more of a heel strike – see pages 18–19). Running toward your forefeet can reduce impact forces and boost your speed.
- Particularly when running at speed, your heels should come up close to your bottom during the recovery phase, although do not over-emphasise this – it should occur naturally.

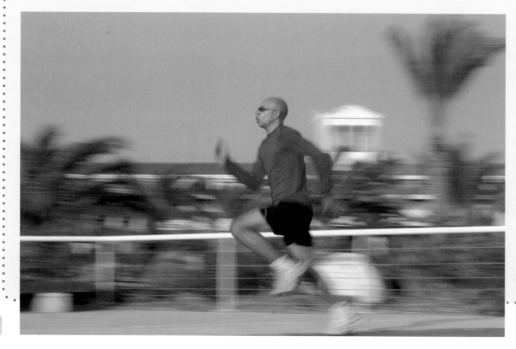

**Good running posture**

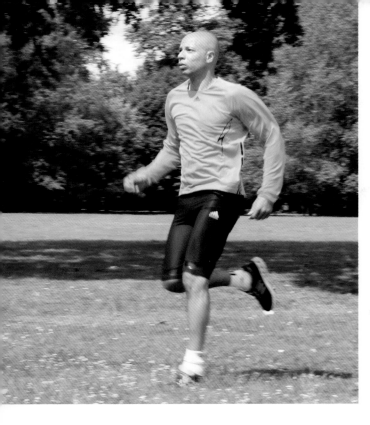

specialist running stores offer foot scans and will recommend the most suitable shoes for you.

Improving your foot-strike will improve your running performance. These drills will "teach" you to strike straighter and more to the front of your foot, which has been shown to reduce impact and therefore potential injury, and also to speed up your running (see page 19).

**The foot-strike/stance phase**

# Ex 3.1 Straight leg jumps

### Benefits
The ankles and calf muscles provide much of the power to the running stride, but runners often overlook them compared to the thighs and glute muscles (the Achilles tendons in particular store and return considerable elastic energy). If you improve their elastic properties through plyometric (jumping) drills, then you can achieve greater speed and distance travelled on each and every stride.

### How to perform
Using only a slight knee bend, jump into the air using your feet and ankles to supply most of the power. Land on your forefeet and immediately launch into another jump. Keep your head and chest up and look straight ahead. Swing your arms backwards and forwards in time with your jump to boost your power.

*Do: 3 x 20 reps*

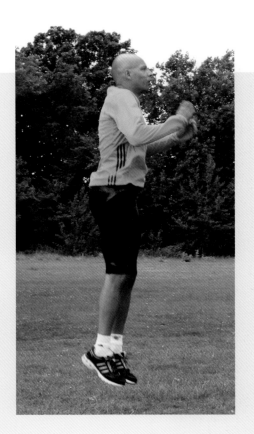

# Ex 3.2 Single leg strike drill

### How to perform

Stand with feet shoulder-width apart and then step forward, lifting one leg out in front of your body to about a 45-degree angle to the ground. Then, keeping the heel up, pull the foot quickly back to the ground. Skip between each "hit". Repeat this "hit", "skip", "hit", "skip" movement, keeping your trunk upright and chin up, while co-ordinating your arms with your legs (that's opposite arm to leg).

*Do: 4 x 20m (swapping legs after each rep)*

### Progression

- Perform the drill with increasing speed and force, skipping more quickly between strikes.
- Perform left, right, left (i.e. alternate foot strikes).

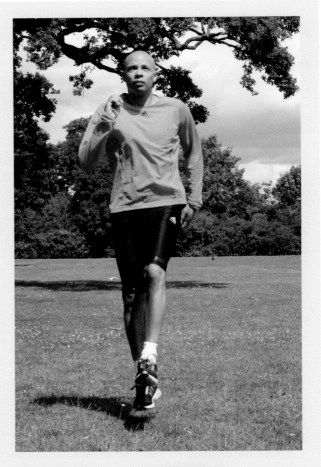

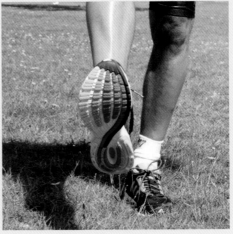

## Ex 3.3 Straight leg bounds

**How to perform**
Stand with your feet about shoulder-width apart and swing one leg to about a 45-degree angle to the ground. Drive it down quickly so that your foot contacts the ground on your forefoot. Immediately "scissor" the other leg up and then down to "pull" yourself forward. Keep your chest elevated and co-ordinate your arms with your legs as you progress over the 20m distance, using what is a type of goose stepping action. The harder you strike the ground, the quicker you will move and the greater the level of the plyometric response.

*Do: 3 x 20m*

**Progression**
After 15m start running normally, while emphasising foot-strike.

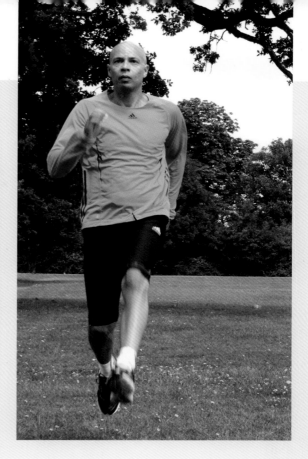

## Ex 3.4 Foot/ground/reaction and recovery phase
This drill can be performed separately on one leg or alternating left and right.

**How to perform**
This description applies to the unilateral (one leg) variant, with the right leg being worked. Start to jog and push the left leg forward, keeping the leg relatively straight, then pull the heel of the right leg dynamically up towards your bottom and through to the front of the hips and then down to strike the ground in a dorsiflexed position (as described in exercise 3.3). Aim to pull your heel back quickly and under your hips to pull you forward, while "spinning" the heel up towards, round and under your body (doing this specifically will improve the recovery phase and develop appropriate hip and hamstring strength in particular). Co-ordinate your arms with your legs – that's opposite arm to leg – and increase the speed of performance as your confidence and specific strength develops. Basically, each leg performs an emphasised leg cycle.

*Do: 4 x 20m (2 on the left and 2 on the right side)*

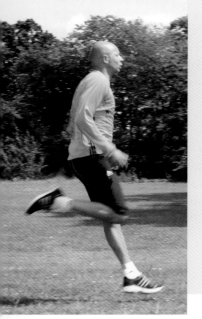

## What is a plyometric action?

A plyometric muscular action is a bit like pulling out a spring and then letting it go – immense amounts of energy will be released as the spring recoils. When you run or jump, the muscles of the ankles, knees and hips are stretched on foot strike when running/landing from the jump (the eccentric contraction). They then fire rapidly as they shorten to produce power (the concentric contraction). Improving your plyometric ability will make you a better runner (plyometric training is covered in more detail in chapter 8).

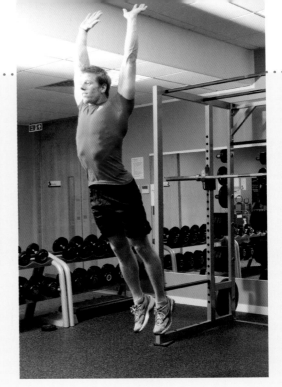

## Recovery phase drills

The recovery phase of the running action takes place after the stance phase, when one foot is on the ground under your hips and it then leaves the ground to be pulled up and through to the front of your body and into the next stride.

Your hamstrings play a vital role in this phase as they contribute to lifting your heel up behind your body and then control its forward momentum once the foot moves to an in-front-of-the-hips position. They then pull the foot back toward the ground in readiness for foot-strike. It's at this point when the hamstring is performing a "lengthening under load" eccentric muscular action. If the hamstring muscles are not eccentrically robust, then strains may occur. The drills that follow are especially suited to developing this particular requirement of hamstring strength (see page 3 for more information).

**The recovery phase**

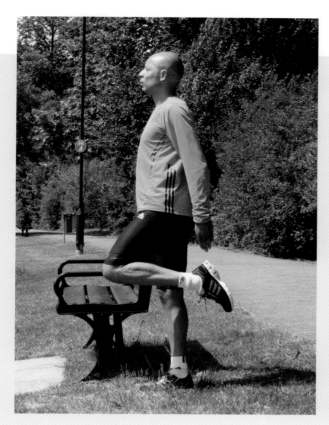

## Ex 3.5 'Four' drill

### How to perform

Stand next to a rail (or suitable height object) and place your inside hand against it for balance. Position your outside leg's foot slightly in advance of the other with the heel slightly lifted off the ground and toes on the ground. Your other (standing) foot should be flat on the ground. Keeping your torso upright, your chest up and gazing straight ahead, use your hamstrings to pull your heel up to your bottom. Your knee will advance in front of your hips at the end position. Don't swing the leg. It's the end position which, when viewed from the side, looks like a "four" – hence the name of the drill. Focus all your energy on "firing" your hamstrings, to pull your heel up and back. For more information on muscle firing see page 64, chapter 6).

*Do: 3 x 10 on each leg*

## Ex 3.6 Single leg cycling

### How to perform

Stand tall – use a rail or other suitable height object for balance. Lift your outside thigh to a position parallel to the ground. Next, sweep the leg down, using your hip flexors (the muscles at the top front of your leg/hip) and round, dynamically pulling your heel up towards your bottom and then bringing it to the front of your hips, before sweeping it back down to the ground again. Increase speed as confidence and specific strength develops.

*Do: 3 x 10 on each leg*

### Progression

Perform two straight legs swings for every cycle.

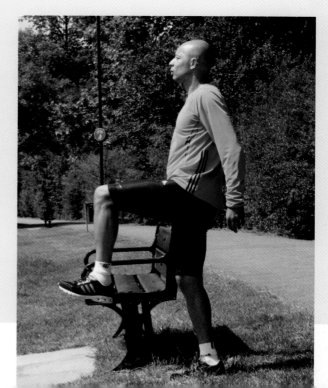

## Ex 3.7 Running leg cycling on the spot

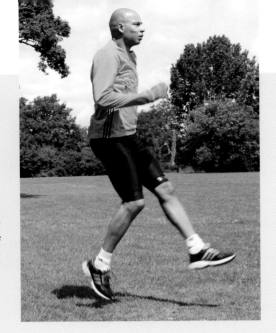

### How to perform
From standing, lift one leg so that its thigh is parallel to the ground, then extend your foreleg and sweep it down to the ground and under your hips, while simultaneously pulling the heel of the other leg up towards your bottom and then through to the front. Co-ordinate your arms with your legs and keep your chest elevated and do not lean back. Repeat this combination of movements. Land on your forefeet and keep your hips pushed forward (don't sit back). Basically you are running on the spot.

*Do: 4 x 20 seconds*

## Ex 3.8 Running leg cycling moving forwards

### How to perform
Begin to jog and then start to cycle each leg so that your ankle passes close to or over the line of the knee of your other leg. Don't lean back to lift your knees – if you are unable to perform the exercise without leaning back, don't lift your knees beyond the point at which leaning back occurs. With practice and through the development of the relevant strength and co-ordination you'll be able to perform the drill correctly. Co-ordinate your arms with your legs, keep your chest elevated and look straight ahead.

*Do: 4 x 20m*

### Tip
Focus on pulling your foot back (keeping your toes dorsiflexed) under your hips dynamically to pull you forwards rapidly over and into each stride.

### Progression
After 10m, gradually extend each leg cycle so that you begin to run more normally – but focus on foot-strike and rotation of the legs on each stride.

## Drive phase drills

The greater the force exerted against the running surface, the faster the speed that will be generated. The "leg drive" is crucial in this respect. This occurs when the grounded leg extends to push you forwards after foot strike and it ends in toe-off, i.e. with your ankles extended. As we've seen, it's actually best to avoid over-emphasising the leg drive as this can often lead to the hips dropping and a loping type of running stride. You'll also expend more energy. However, by performing specific leg drive drills you will increase your propulsion and therefore your running speed. "Drive drills" are highly relevant to improving acceleration.

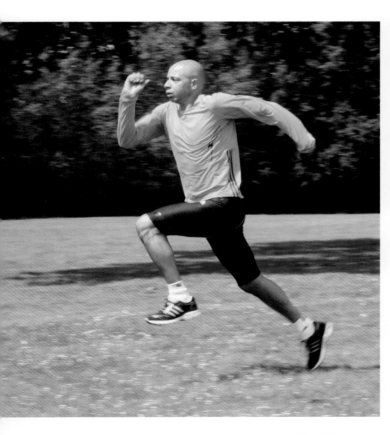

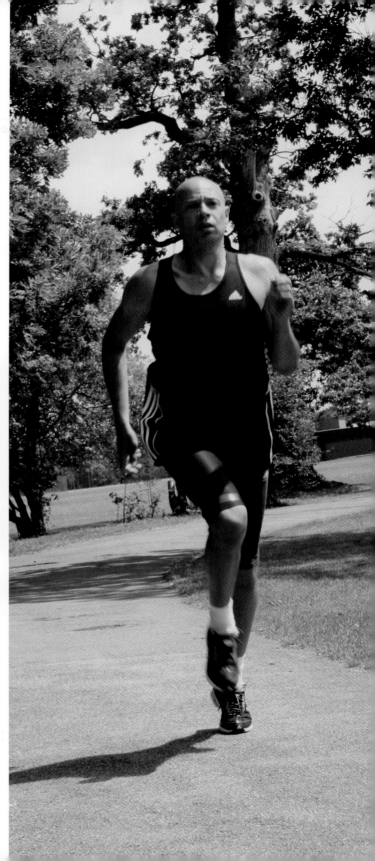

**The drive phase**

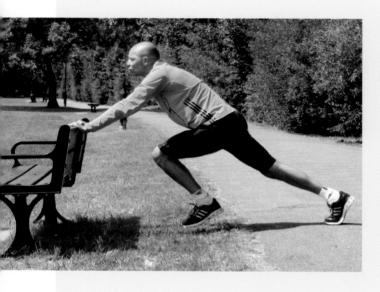

## Ex 3.9 Stationary wall leg drives

**How to perform**
Stand facing a wall (or similar object) with your hands against it. Walk your feet back so that your body is leaning into the wall in a straight line of about 45 degrees. Lift one thigh so that it is at right angles to your hips and your lower leg is at right angles to your knee. Next, drive your foot dynamically back towards the ground to strike it slightly behind your standing foot and then dynamically lift it to return to the start position. Brace your core throughout. Perform the designated number of reps and then swap sides.

*Do: 3 x 10 reps (on each leg)*

## Ex 3.10 Speed bounds

**How to perform**
Mark out a distance of 20m on a suitable surface, such as a running track, or dry flat grass. Start with your legs hip-width apart. Lift one thigh parallel to the ground and then dynamically drive the leg behind you to push yourself forward, pulling the other to the fore, so that its thigh is parallel to the ground. Then, without extending the foot of this leg too far in advance of the knee, bring it back down to the ground in a piston-like action, to perform another drive. Continue "driving" over the ground to complete the 20m distance, focusing on pushing yourself horizontally and not vertically all the while. Keep your toes up (dorsiflexed) on each foot strike and try to make each contact as light and as quick as you can. Co-ordinate your arms with your legs and don't look down.

*Do: 4 x 20m*

**Progression**
After 15m begin to run normally.

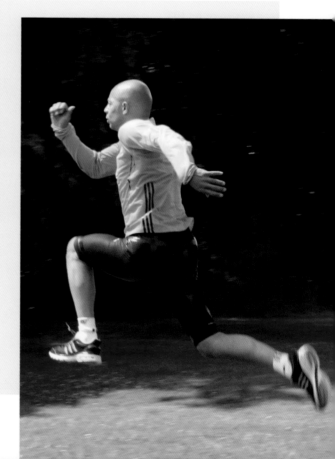

## Arm action drills

If you are a recreational runner, you don't need to pump your arms like Usain Bolt when on a long run. However, whatever your speed, a powerful yet relaxed arm drive and carriage will increase your speed potential. (Note a powerful arm action is needed for faster running and sprinting – of which more in chapter 6).

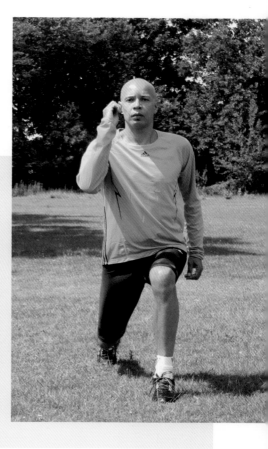

### Ex 3.11 Lunge position sprint arm action

**How to perform**

Take a large step forward into a lunge. Both knees should be bent to 90 degrees. Keep the knee of your front leg over its ankle and the knee of the rear leg a few centimetres from the floor. With your chest elevated, drive your arms backwards and forwards as if sprinting. Maintain a 90-degree angle at your elbows and your shoulders square onto the front, chin parallel to the ground and eyes looking forward throughout. Your hands should reach a position in line with your eyes to the front of your body with upper arms parallel to the floor behind. You will move your arms faster if you do not "force" the movement and remain relaxed.

*Do: 4 x 30 seconds with a 60-second recovery (2 sets each with a right and left leg lunge lead)*

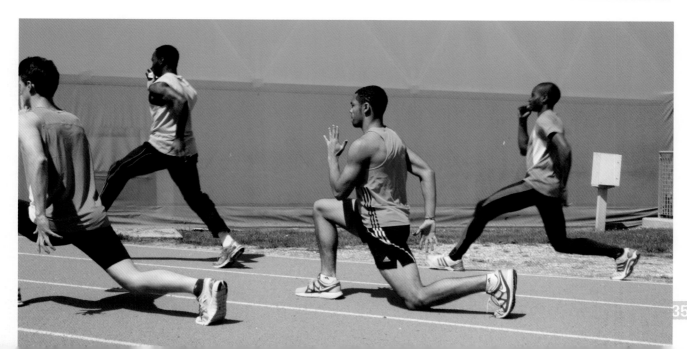

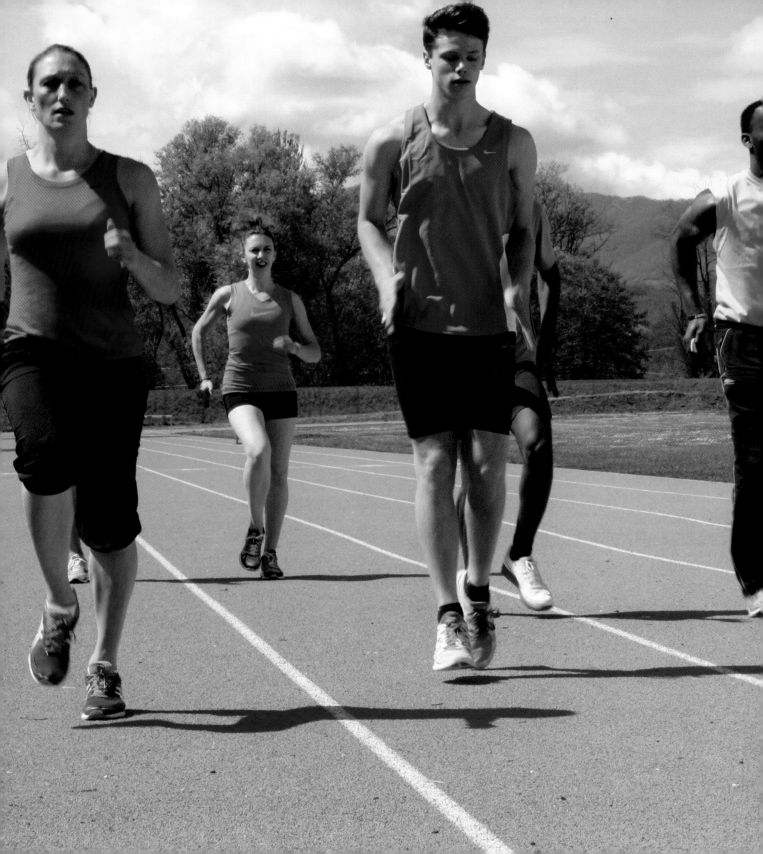

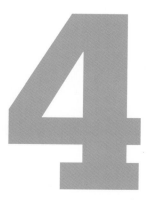

# running-specific warm-ups

The approach to warming up for sports activities has changed dramatically in recent years. Traditionally warms-ups would involve 5–15 minutes of gentle cardiovascular exercise to raise body temperature, usually jogging, followed by static (held) stretches. There are much more effective ways to warm up for all sports and this includes running.

Many of the exercises mentioned in chapters 1 and 2 are also suitable for inclusion in your running warm-ups, for example, leg cycling. You should build up a repertoire of warm-up routines that include combinations of the various exercises described in this book.

## The sports-specific warm-up

The sports-specific warm-up probably originated from the former Soviet Bloc (particularly for speed and power athletes). Their athletes were using these types of warm-ups from at least the 1970s, but it is only relatively recently that they have become popular in the West. The sports-specific warm-up is designed to optimally prepare body and mind for sport. It is focused and progressively dynamic. This means that the pace of the exercises and drills that you perform build in terms of their speed and power requirements across the warm-up.

Exercise physiologists have often challenged the physical value of a warm-up – some suggested that in real terms there is little actual value to it. However, for an athlete from any sport to enter a competitive or training situation without prior preparation seems inconceivable. The rationale behind the running/ sports-specific warm-up is at least a much stronger one, when compared with the older traditional warm-up format. However, as a runner you might think that a gentle jog before commencing your faster run is all that is needed. Yes, you could probably get away with this, however, by not warming up more extensively you are missing out on a prime opportunity to strengthen your running muscles and perform drills and exercises that will boost your performance over time and reduce your risk of injury.

## Why warm up specifically for running?

A running-specific warm-up will:

- raise body temperature – this process will "switch on" numerous physiological processes that make subsequent vigorous exercise more effective and safer;
- get you mentally ready to exercise, by putting you in the right frame of mind to get the best from your body (known to sports psychologists as being in the "zone of optimal functioning" or simply "in the zone");
- boost your neuromuscular system so, should you be competing, you are better placed to do so (of which more later and particularly relevant to sprinters and fast short-distance interval training);
- improve specific range of movement – muscles literally become more stretchy (as body temperature increases and muscle fibres prepare for more dynamic movements);

## Static stretches

There will be some runners out there that feel you need to perform held stretches as part of your warm-up. If you can, I'd recommend that you gradually reduce their input into your warm-ups in favour of the active, more specific approach discussed in this chapter. Aim to only perform static stretches as a peripheral element to your running warm-up. They could be used, for example, to elongate muscles that are prone to tightness during your workouts, for example, the calf muscles. It is important to realise that held types of stretches have little actual value in terms of improving running performance, in fact they can be detrimental, as they reduce the elasticity of your muscles. However, static stretches do have a place to play in your running training routines (see page 49).

## Cool-downs

It is important to cool down after a run. The process will return your body to more of a steady state, winding down the elevated physiological responses created by running. A cool-down will specifically reduce the build-up of lactate (lactic acid) and help to ease out potential residual muscle soreness.

Lactate is a chemical that is present in the body at all times and is a key constituent of muscular action, and its levels of production increase with exercise. At higher intensities its chemical structure will alter and it then becomes lactic acid. Lactic acid results in burning muscles and pain! Cooling down will help to reduce the build-up of lactic acid and return lactate levels to nearer normal levels.

- increase oxygen use in muscles, as haemoglobin* release is facilitated at higher body temperatures – the warmer the body, the better the haemoglobin release;
- enhance your progressive development of running-specific strength, through using running-specific exercises;
- improve your running technique by the regular and progressive performance of specific running exercises; and
- increase your speed – due to a combination of all of the above!

* Haemoglobin is the major element of red blood cells. It is an iron/protein compound that boosts the oxygen carrying ability of blood by about 65 times.

# Running-specific warm-up exercises

The exercises described in the following section are applicable to runners of all speeds and abilities. Jog for a minimum of 5 minutes before performing them and progress gradually in terms of distance, reps and sets (the drills covered in the previous two chapters can also be included). Suggested reps and sets are provided but these are for guideline purposes only.

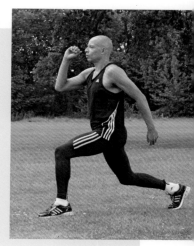

## Ex 4.1 Lunge walk

**Benefits**
This exercise loosens up the hips and hamstrings and strengthens the quads, glutes and hamstring muscles.

**How to perform**
Take a large step forward into a lunge then step forward into another lunge. Keep your chest up and look straight ahead, co-ordinating arm and leg movements (opposite arm to leg). Keep your knee behind your ankle when planting on each lunge.

*Do: 4 x 20m*

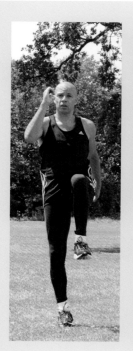
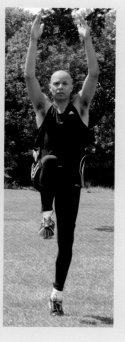

## Ex 4.2 High knee march

**Benefits**
This exercise benefits the hip flexor muscles and ankle strength and improves the running drive phase.

**How to perform**
Extend onto the toes of one leg, while lifting the thigh parallel to the ground. Next, dynamically drive this leg towards the ground to strike it on your forefoot, while lifting the other to a thigh's parallel position. Repeat. Co-ordinate your arms with your legs and keep the chest elevated throughout. The speed of the drill can be increased as the warm-up progresses.

*Do: 4 x 15m*

**Progressions**
Perform with arms held straight over head (see photo) or perform holding a Powerbag or weights disc at arm's length.

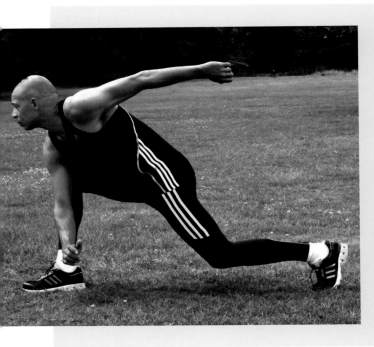

## Ex 4.3 Elbow to inside of ankle lunge

### Benefits
This exercise benefits hip flexibility and hamstring strength and will also develop better balance. The forward lean also stretches the lower back.

### How to perform
This exercise is very similar to exercise 4.1, the lunge walk, except that you should extend your trunk forwards over your extended leg during each lunge. So, if your right leg were to the front, you would take your right elbow down to the inside of your right ankle. Pause, then step into another lunge, incline your trunk forward and repeat to the left side.

*Do: 4 x 15m*

## Ex 4.4 Calf drill

### Benefits
This exercise benefits lower limb and Achilles tendon strength and flexibility.

### How to perform
Keep your legs relatively straight and use a heel-to-toe action to move forward. Co-ordinate your arms with your legs and keep your chest elevated. Try to "roll" across each foot and take small steps.

*Do: 4 x 20m*

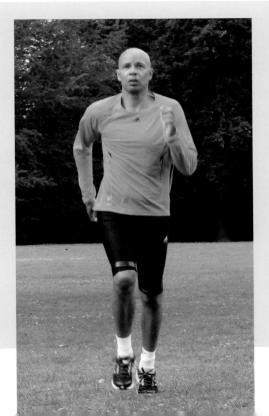

## Ex 4.5 Backwards running

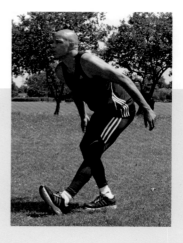

### Benefits
This exercise benefits lower limb and ankle strength, agility and flexibility. Also known as back-pedals, they are often used by sports rehabilitation specialists treating ACL injuries (see chapter 1) and lower back injuries. Often the injured runner can back pedal before they can run forwards.

### How to perform
A great warm-up exercise, performing drills such as backwards running will also pre-condition against common running injuries, such as shin-splints, and strengthen the knee and ankle joints. While doing them you should focus on being "light" on your feet and generating movement from the balls of your feet. This plyometric drill will improve your reactivity and leg power.

*Do: 3–4 x 20m*

### Progressions
On pushing back into each step, lift each leg up, out and back further, to run in reverse. This will open up stride length and develop quadriceps and calf muscle strength.

## Ex 4.6 Simulated running arm action
See page 35 for details on how to perform this exercise.

## Ex 4.7 Hamstring and lower back walk and sweep stretch

### Benefits
This exercise will mobilise your lower back and hamstrings, which is an area in which runners often suffer from stiffness/tightness.

### How to perform
Step forwards, placing the heel of your extended leg on the ground and dorsiflexing your foot, while sitting back over your rear leg's heel and sweeping your arms from behind your body to a position in front. Hold for a split second and then stand and move forward by advancing the rear leg to the front and repeating the movement. If you experience problems, isolate one rep at a time, performing a number of reps to one side at a time.

*Do: 4 x 10 reps*

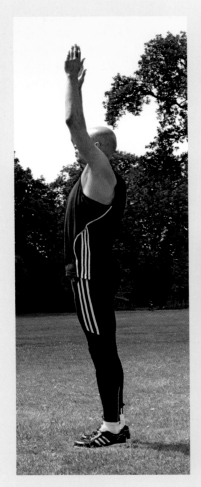

# Ex 4.8 Standing to press-up

### Benefits
This exercise warms up the lower back, hamstrings, calf muscles and torso (and also strengthens the latter, the shoulders and the chest).

### How to perform
Stand tall and hinge from your hips to place your fingers/hands (depending on your flexibility) on the ground in front of your feet. Then gradually start to walk your hands away from you, extending your body into a press-up position as you do so. Complete a designated number of press-ups and then walk your hands back in to stand back up.

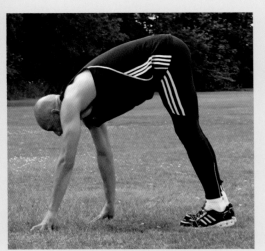

*Do: 6 reps*

### Progressions
Make the press-ups strong – lower to a two count and press up to a one count.

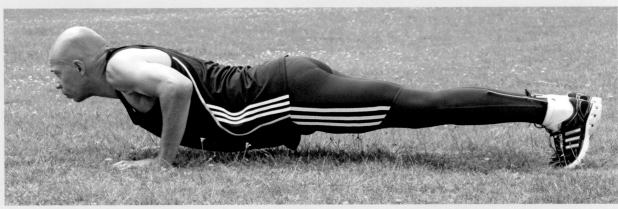

## Maximise your warm-up – stretch and strengthen

Many of the warm-up exercises and drills described serve a number of functions. Exercise 4.8, the standing to press-up drill, is a prime example, acting as both a dynamic mobility exercise and a strengthening one for the core and upper body. Some may argue that these exercises, particularly of the type shown in this chapter, should be performed only in specific workouts away from running sessions. However, to do this is to miss a valuable point: the inclusion of such exercises in your warm-up provides a double whammy that can maximise your running strength development and training time.

A further example of such an exercise is the plank with leg raise.

## Ex 4.9 Plank with leg raise

### Benefits
This exercise strengthens the core and warms up the hips and hamstrings.

### How to perform
Assume a plank position (see exercise 8.19, page 108), supporting your weight on your forearms and toes. Hold the plank position for 10 seconds and then gently lift and lower one leg at a time for 10 reps.

*Do: 3–6 reps*

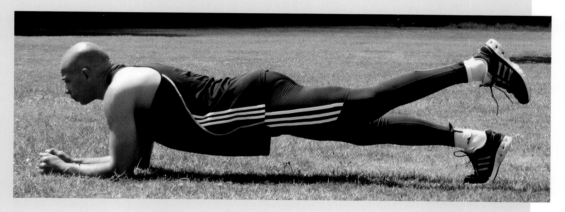

## The relevance of stretching to running

Despite the relevance to enhanced performance of a running-specific warm-up and using the drills described in previous chapters, there is still a place for stretching in your training.

As a runner you will be familiar with static held (active/passive-type) stretches, such as bending down to the toes, to stretch the hamstrings. These may have formed the mainstay of your running warm-ups in the past, however, they actually have little relevance to specifically preparing your body for running. Despite this, there is still a need to incorporate them and other similar styles of stretching into your running training for the following reasons:

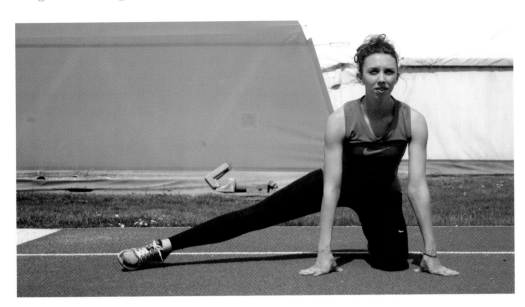

Stretching does have a place in your running warm-up and cool-down.

- **To improve/maintain running/sport-specific range of movement.** If you have tight hamstrings, quadriceps and hip muscles, you will be more prone to injury, such as "runner's knee" (see chapter 1, page 5).
- **To aid relaxation and recovery.** Because of the dynamic nature of running, training can tighten muscles. Regular stretching will combat this tightness and aid recovery.
- **To boost the effectiveness of the cool-down.** As a runner you should stretch as part of your cool-down to aid recovery and elongate muscles that may have tightened during their workout (note: if you have performed a very intense workout, then your muscles will have lost some of their elasticity and will be overly fatigued – when that happens, only light stretches (comfortable) should be performed).

Stretching and its relevance to running is covered in detail in chapter 5.

# Foam rollers and massage sticks

Relatively recently foam rollers and massage sticks have become mainstream for everyday sportsmen and sportswomen and fitness trainers. Their function is to warm up muscles and to re-align muscle fibres and boost recovery by "rolling out" muscle soreness. I'd recommend that you add one to your training kit. Apply light pressure at first and then increase gradually. If you use this tool as part of your warm-up, do not apply "very painful pressure". Away from your workouts – and used as a means to promote recovery from sore muscles – greater pressure can be used.

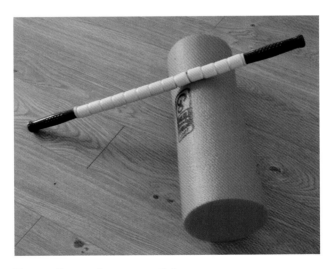

Foam rollers and massage sticks

## Sample foam roller exercises

Perform each exercise 2–3 times for 30 seconds each.

### Ex 4.10 Front of the thighs (quads)

**How to perform**

In a plank position (see exercise 8.19, page 108) and with the foam roller under your thighs, position your body weight so that it is supported on your elbows, then place one leg across the other so that one leg takes all the weight. Move yourself up and down so that the roller massages your thighs. Change legs.

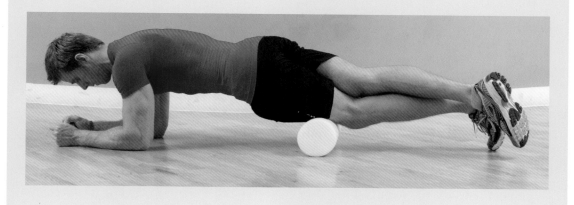

### Ex 4.11 ITB (illiotibial band)

**How to perform**

Lie on your side with the foam roller under your left thigh. Support your weight with your forearms/hand. Stack your feet on top of each other, then position your right leg in front of the left with your instep on the floor, with your knee bent. Roll across the roller, stopping whenever you reach a tender spot. You can increase the intensity by stacking your legs.

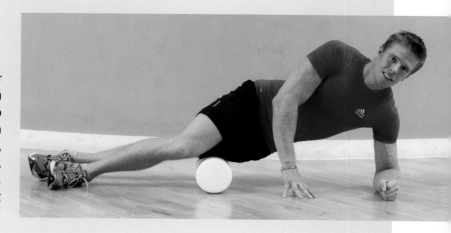

## Ex 4.12 Back of the thighs (hamstrings)

**How to perform**
Sit on the ground and place the foam roller under your thighs. Support your weight through your arms. Roll forwards and backwards so the roller moves from your bottom to your knees. To work one leg more intensely cross your legs over as in the bottom image.

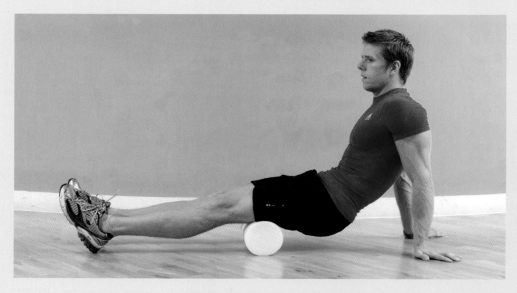

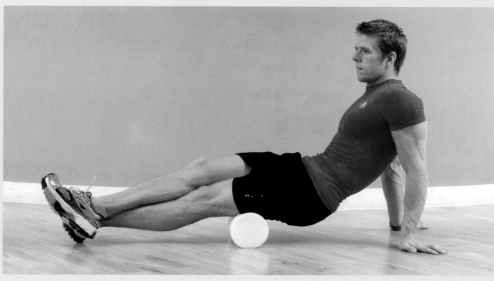

# Ex 4.13 Calf muscles (gastrocnemius and soleus)

### How to perform

Sit with your legs extended and place the foam roller under your calfs. Put your hands behind you to support your torso. Roll backwards and forwards across the roller so that it moves from your ankle to your knee.

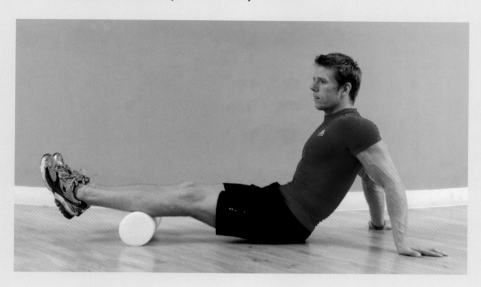

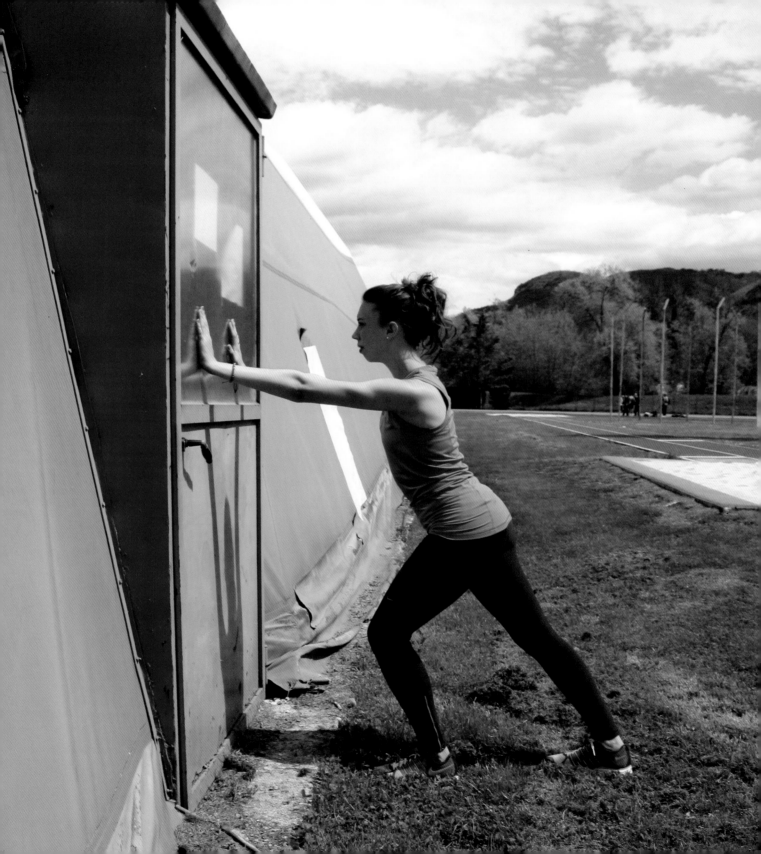

# 5 running and stretching

Although the focus of this book is obviously on strength training, it would be remiss not to provide some information on stretching and some specific stretches that you can do away from your running and strength training sessions to maintain specific mobility and promote recovery. This section also includes information on related subjects such as Pilates. Pilates is now very popular among the general fitness population, sportsmen and sportswomen and runners. It's a great way to promote flexibility, strength, balance and postural awareness.

Static (held) type stretches have little direct benefit to enhancing running performance. Running takes muscles through dynamic ranges of movement whereas a passive stretch, such as bending forward from your hips to touch your toes, while keeping your legs straight, to stretch your hamstrings, does not. Research into running and other sports such as rugby and football has actually indicated that passive stretching, in particular during the warm-up, may be connected to hamstring strain at a more serious level and reduced performance at a lower one (see panel on the next page).

However, as has been shown, stretching does have a role to play in your running conditioning programme, as it helps you to recover from sessions and maintain your running-specific range of mobility. The lower back, hips, hamstrings, quadriceps, calf muscles, shoulders and Achilles tendons will all benefit from regular focused stretching.

## Factors affecting flexibility

### Gender

As a general rule, women tend to be more flexible than men. This is due to the physiological differences between the sexes, in particular specific hormone levels. Women produce more of the hormone relaxin, which is essential for pregnancy and childbirth. Relaxin does as it sounds – it relaxes muscles and makes them more elastic.

### Your age

Age also affects flexibility. Muscles and joints become stiffer with age, hence it's more important for older runners to maintain a stretching regime, which will not only benefit running, but will also help to combat ageing. It's worth noting that range of movement can be increased whatever our age by dedicating "stretch time" (see chapter 11).

## Running stretches

Perform these stretches in a warm environment 2–3 times a week, preferably on days when you are not training (or 3–4 hours after a workout). A good time to stretch is after you have had a hot bath or shower, as your muscles will be relaxed and your core temperature elevated, making stretching easier. Where appropriate, hold each stretch for 20–30 seconds and repeat 2–3 times (if you stretch during warm-up, do not go for maximum stretches and hold only for 10 seconds), then perform a selection of drills from chapter 4 after your stretches. These take your muscles dynamically through ranges of movement which are similar to those involved in running.

## Stretching in the warm-up does not enhance performance

Many runners believe that stretching will get them ready to run better than they would if they had not stretched during a warm-up, however, the majority of research indicates that pre-running stretching can actually impair performance.

Researchers looked into the effects of static stretching on the energy expended by endurance runners. Ten male runners aged 25 participated in the research. Their VO$_2$max indicated an above average level of ability. The runners performed three tests. Firstly, their anthropometrics (body measurements) and VO$_2$max were measured (VO$_2$max indicates the maximum oxygen processing ability of an athlete – the higher it is the greater the lung capacity. Although VO$_2$max responds to training, its ability is largely inherited. Once calculated by means of, usually, a lab test, percentages of VO$_2$max can be exercised at in order to 'control' energy expenditure). Then, separated by a week, the runners performed a 60 minute treadmill run – one was preceded by stretching and the other was not. Stretching consisted of 16 minutes of static stretching using five exercises for the major lower body muscle groups. For the non-stretching protocol the runners sat quietly for 16 minutes. The run involved a 30 minute effort at 65 per cent of VO$_2$max followed by a 30 minute "performance run" where participants ran as far as possible without viewing distance or speed. Total calories expended were determined for the 30 minutes at 65 per cent VO$_2$max, while distance covered provided the determinant for the performance run. The researchers discovered that the non-stretching runners performed better during the 65 per cent VO$_2$max effort. In terms of calories burned they achieved 425 (+/- 50) vs. 405 (+/- 50) kcals. This level of superior performance was also displayed in the performance run: the non-stretching runners completed an average of 6.0km (+/- 1.1 km), as opposed to the stretching runners who achieved an average of (5.8km (+/- 1.0 km). This led the researchers to conclude that "stretching before an endurance event may lower endurance performance and increase the energy cost of running."[1]

## Ex 5.1 Hip flexor stretch

**Targets**
This stretch targets the hip flexors.

**How to perform**
Assume a kneeling lunge position, with your trunk elevated and chin parallel to the ground and hands on the front of your thigh. Position yourself so that you feel a stretch in the top of your thighs/hip region. Gently push your hip forwards and slide your rear leg backwards to extend the stretch.

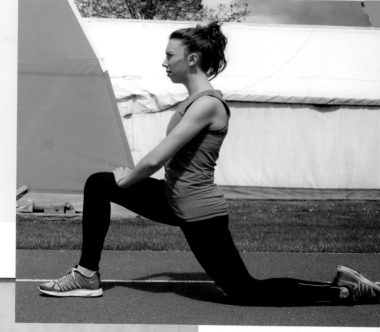

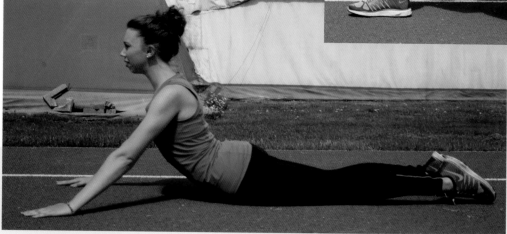

## Ex 5.2 Cobra (hyper-extension)

**Targets**
This stretch targets the abdominals.

**How to perform**
Lie on your front with your hands near or under your shoulders. Extend your arms to lift your chest off the floor. Keep your hips in contact with the ground.

## Ex 5.3 Quad stretch

### Targets
This stretch targets the quads.

### How to perform
Stand on one leg and pull the heel of the unsupported leg up toward your bottom by grasping the top of your foot. Point your knee down to the ground and try to keep your torso upright and your gaze straight ahead. Hold and repeat on both sides. This stretch can also be performed from a lying on your side position.

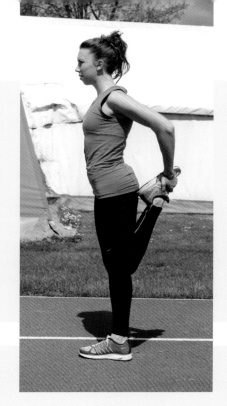

## Ex 5.4 Illiotibial band (ITB) stretch

### Targets
This stretch targets the ITB.

### How to perform
The ITB is an area of fascia that runs over the muscles of the outer portion of the thigh (fascia is a type of soft issue that covers muscles, binding some together and allowing others to move). With repeated running it can become tight and place a strain on the structures of the knee – specifically "runner's knee" (see page 5). Stretching the ITB can be difficult; however, one of the best ways to do this is by lying on your back. Bend the leg that doesn't need to be stretched at the knee, keeping your foot flat on the ground. Then hook the leg of the ITB band to be stretched over the thigh of the bended leg. Place your hands behind the bended leg and control the stretch by pulling the supporting thigh in towards you using your hip muscles and hands. Hold and repeat on both sides.

Runners who suffer from "runner's knee" often have weak hip abductor muscles – see chapters 8 and 9 for relevant glute medius strengthening exercises, which will help to ease this.

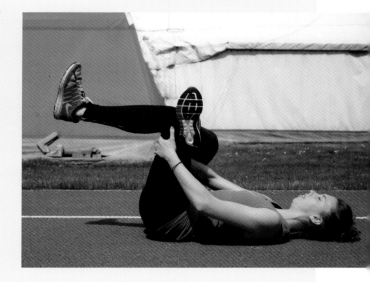

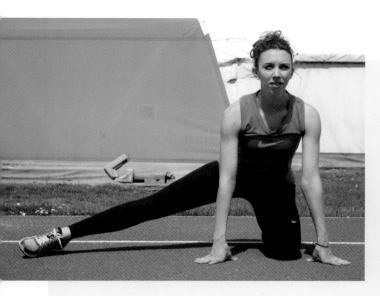

## Ex 5.5 Kneeling adductor stretch

**Targets**
This stretch targets the adductors (inside of the thighs).

**How to perform**
Kneel and lean forwards, placing your hands on the floor for support. Extend one leg straight out to the side, your thighs should be level. Slide your straight leg away until you feel a stretch in your inner thigh area. Do not allow your back to excessively round.

## Ex 5.6 Front lying lower back, hip flexor and quadriceps stretch

**Targets**
This stretch targets the lower back, hip flexor and quadriceps.

**How to perform**
Lie on your front with your hands outstretched in a chest down crucifix position. Keeping one leg pressed into the floor lift the other leg up and attempt to reach its foot across to its opposite hand, rotating your hips and lower back to do so and allowing the knee to bend. Hold the stretch for 10 seconds and then return the leg to the start position. Try to keep your chest on the floor at all times. Repeat on the other side.

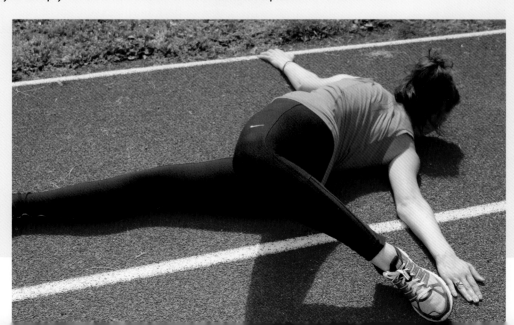

## Ex 5.7 Glute stretch

**Targets**
This stretch targets the glutes.

**How to perform**
Lie on your back and clasp your hands just below the knee of one leg, having pulled it in towards you. Keep the other leg flat on the floor. Keeping your upper body on the ground, gently pull your knee in towards your chest. Keep your head on the ground.

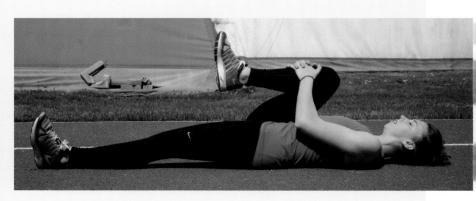

## Ex 5.8 Calf stretch (gastrocnemius)

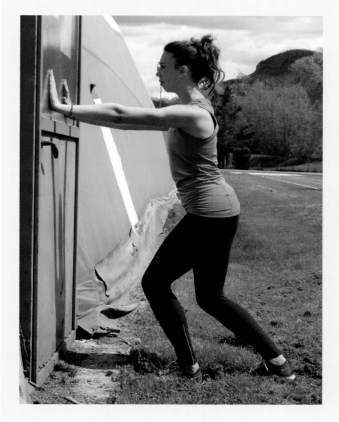

**Targets**
This stretch targets the calf muscles.

**How to perform**
Stand close to a wall and place your hands against it at shoulder level and at arm's length. Step one foot back and press your heel into the ground to specifically stretch the calf muscles, the gastrocnemius. Hold the stretch for 10 seconds, step back to the start position and repeat with the other leg.

## Ex 5.9 Calf and Achilles tendon stretch

### Targets
This stretch targets the soleus and Achilles tendon.

### How to perform
Stand on a low ledge. Drop your heel back and down towards the ground. Hold this position to stretch your Achilles tendons in particular.

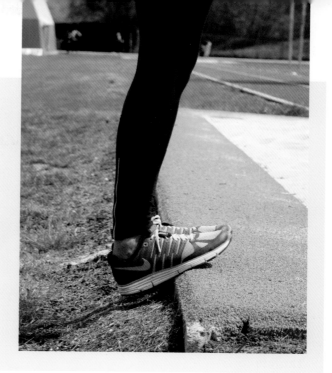

## Ex 5.10 Hamstring stretch

### Targets
This stretch targets the hamstrings.

### How to perform
Stand with your feet together. Take a small step backwards with one leg and then bend your rear knee so that your thighs are parallel. Push your hips back and with chest up and lower back slightly hinged, bend forward. Place your hands on your bent leg for support. You can also pull your toes up on your leading foot to stretch your gastrocnemius.

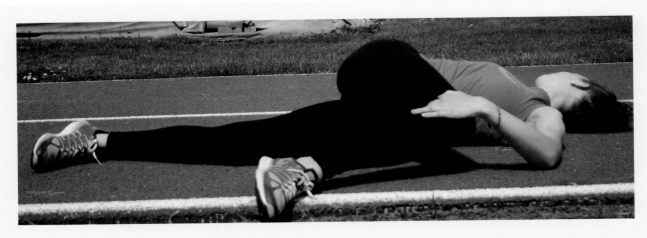

## Ex 5.11 Obliques stretch

**Targets**

This stretch targets the obliques (outer core muscles, hips and shoulders).

**How to perform**

Lie on your back with your legs straight and your arms extended out to the side so you form a "T" shape. Bend one leg and place your foot flat on the floor. Then reach across and place your opposite hand on your knee. Pull your knee over and rotate your lower body while keeping your other arm outstretched and shoulders flat on the ground. Hold this position allowing the weight of your leg, combined with pulling on your knee with your arm, to achieve a deeper stretch.

## Ex 5.12 Shoulder stretch

**Targets**

This stretch targets the shoulders.

**How to perform**

Although a lack of shoulder flexibility is less likely to create injuries, it is important to remain flexible in this area, particularly if you are a sprinter where range of movement as well as power is required. Stand with your feet shoulder-width apart and knees slightly bent. Raise your hands so your palms are facing forwards. Keeping your shoulders pulled together and without arching your lower back, take your arms above your head. Lower your arms until your hands are level with your shoulders.

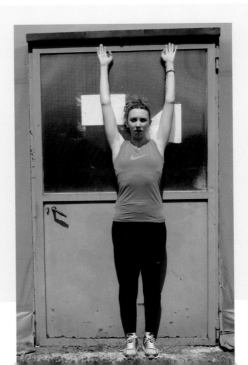

## Ex 5.13 Chest stretch

**Targets**
This stretch targets the chest.

**How to perform**
Stand with your feet shoulder-width apart. Fully extend you arms in front of you with interlocked fingers. Push forward through your shoulders and arms and return to the start.

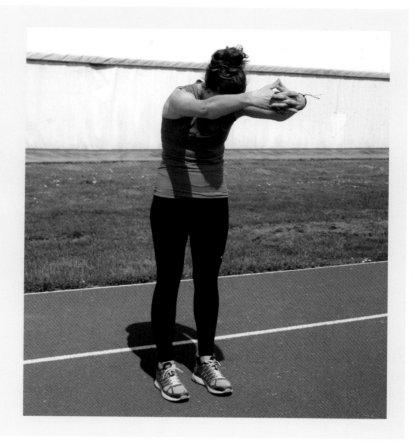

## Different types of stretches
There are several different ways that muscles can be stretched.

### Passive stretches
Those in the above section are what is known as "passive" stretches. During a passive stretch the force used to develop the stretch is applied, for example, by yourself, via another person, through the use of stretch bands or by holding onto an object.

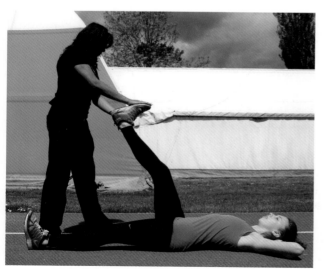

During a passive stretch the force to stretch a muscle/muscles is supplied externally. This passive stretch shows the hamstrings being stretched.

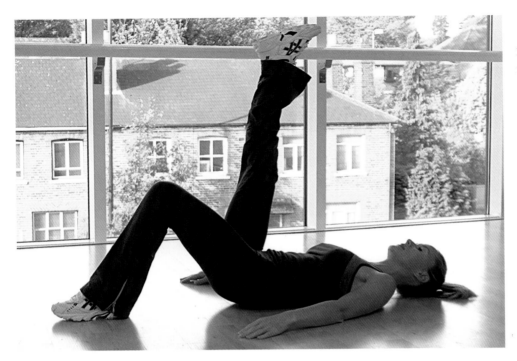

During an active stretch the force required to stretch a muscle/muscles is supplied by yourself.

## Active stretches

An active stretch involves muscles being stretched by you physically moving a limb into position to promote the stretch without external added force. The power behind the stretch is supplied by deliberate muscular action.

As well as maintaining/improving range of movement, active stretches can also develop strength. This is because muscular power is needed to hold the stretched position. A couple of examples of running-specific active stretches are provided below:

### Hamstring active stretch

**How to perform**

Sit on the floor with one leg bent to 90 degrees and your torso supported through bent arms with your forearms on the floor behind your body. Lean back slightly. Lift the other leg, while maintaining a slight bend at the knee back towards your torso to stretch your hamstrings. Pull the leg in as far as you can and hold for 20 seconds. Lower the leg under control and repeat on the other side. This stretch also strengthens your hip flexors.

### Glute active stretch

**How to perform**

Assume the same starting position as for the previous exercise. Bend one knee to a 90-degree angle and then pull the leg in towards your chest using your hip flexor muscles. Hold for the desired duration. Extend the leg back to the start position under control and repeat on the other side. Keep pressing the other leg into the floor.

## Flexibility – is too much a bad thing?

Some research indicates that it is actually possible to be too flexible. Researchers looking into joint flexibility in sub-elite marathon runners indicated that "inflexibility in certain areas of the musculoskeletal system may enhance running economy in sub-elite male runners by increasing storage and return of elastic energy and minimising the need for muscle-stabilising activity."[2] In other words they are saying that a more circumspect approach to developing flexibility as a runner is potentially better than one that strives to develop it extensively. To further substantiate this perspective:

When studying 21 male distance runners, researchers discovered that longer Achilles tendons and less flexible knee and ankle joints made for improved running economy.[3]

## Stretching and recovery – the role of stretching in your cool-down

Stretching after a run as part of a cool-down can promote recovery. Note: If you have performed an intense workout then stretches should be gentle and maximal range (the furthest you can stretch the muscle) avoided. Tired muscles are more prone to injury (see page 38 for more information on the cool-down).

## How flexible do you need to be as a runner?

As we saw in chapter 1, the main need for specific running range of mobility is just that – you should have sufficient range of movement around your joints to be able to run fluently and without strain. If range of mobility is particularly great around a joint, then the joint may be less stable and less "stiff" and less able to generate force – this is particularly so (though not exclusively) for very fast and sprint running, where fast, dynamic and firm movements need to be made. Stretching to improve range of movement is best performed separately to running workouts and should only be performed to maintain running-specific ranges of movement and to promote recovery. Excessive flexibility can be detrimental to run performance.

## Pilates for runners

Pilates, with its emphasis on the core, postural control, breathing and range of movement, can be of use to the runner. Indeed, many professional sports teams and athletes make it a regular feature of their training. Advice is best sourced from a qualified Pilates instructor. Some examples of running-relevant Pilates exercises are provided below.

## Ex 5.14 Side lying leg circles

### Benefits

This exercise strengthens the muscles of the hip and bottom.

### How to perform

Rest on your right side, with your right leg bent in front of you for stability and your left arm folded and positioned on your hip. Extend your left leg and hold it at hip height and

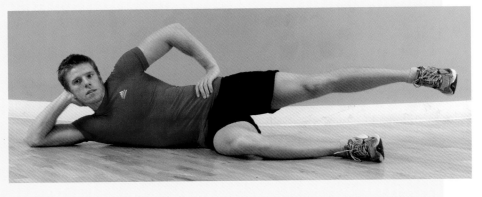

then draw circles in the air 8–10 times in each direction. Keep your hips still and waist lengthened and off the floor throughout. Pause and then repeat on the other side.

*Do: 8–10 reps*

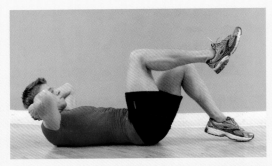

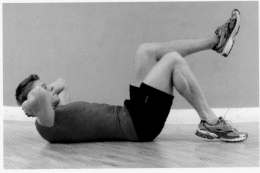

## Ex 5.15 Pilates toe taps

### Benefits

This exercise strengthens and stabilises the core.

### How to perform

Place your hands behind your head and flex your head and shoulders forwards. Breathe in and lift one leg at a time until your knees are above your hips and bent to 90 degrees. Breathe out and lower one foot towards the floor. As you progress, straighten your leg as you lower it, but only lower as far as you can while maintaining neutral spine and a flat stomach.

### Progression

Straighten your leg as you lower it but only do so as far as you can while maintaining a neutral spine and a flat stomach.

*Do: 20 reps*

## PNF stretching

Proprioceptive neuromuscular facilitation (PNF) stretching is often recommended as one of the best ways to improve your range of mobility (note: this should only be undertaken if there is a need for increased range to improve running technique or reduce injury potential). Although it's possible to perform PNF stretches on your own, perhaps with the aid of a towel or a band, it's best to have a partner.

PNF stretching works on the basis of two-directional force increasing the stretch potential of the muscles by "short-circuiting" the stretch reflex. The stretch reflex is a complex mechanism that prevents a muscle from being over stretched. If you were to stretch your hamstrings while lying on your back, keeping the other flat and pulling one leg up and towards you, a point would be reached when the leg would travel no more, which is the result of the stretch reflex kicking in. PNF stretching deactivates the stretch reflex for a short period, so that the stretch can be extended beyond previous limits.

## Ex 5.16 PNF hamstring stretch

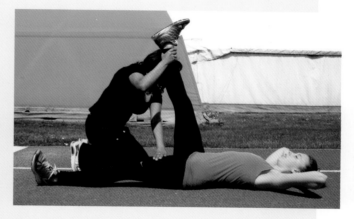

### How to perform

Lie on your back with your arms by your sides. A training partner should assist as you lift one leg up and back towards your head. Maintain a slight bend at the knee joint of the active leg, with the other leg pressed firmly into the ground (your partner can press on this leg with their hand to achieve this). The leg being stretched will travel back to a point where further movement becomes difficult – this is when the stretch reflex activates. This position should be held for 20 seconds. Next, apply force by pushing back against your partner through the leg (your partner must obviously be braced and ready to offer resistance). Relax (i.e. stop pressing) and then press again for a further 15 seconds. Your partner should then be able to gently push your leg into an increased range of movement and hold for a further 10 seconds.

## References

1  *Journal of Strength & Conditioning Research*, 2010 Sep; 24(9):2274

2  *Medicine and Science in Sports and Exercise*, June 1996; 28(6):737-743

3  *Medicine and Science in Sports and Exercise*, August 2011; 43(8),1492-1499

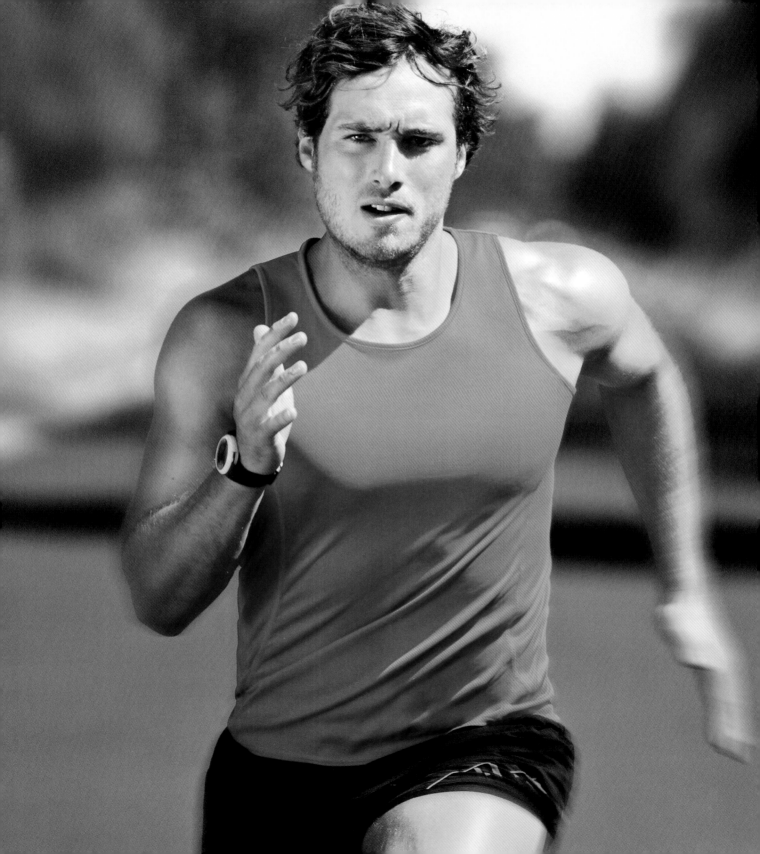

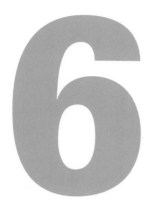

# sprinting for faster and stronger running

Sprinting is obviously a form of running, yet it's not something that many recreational runners do. There are a number of benefits to be made from incorporating some sprinting and sprint work into your training: the faster your top speed, the easier it will be for you to maintain a slower pace, and sprinting is a very specific way of developing greater running strength and power.

There have been various examples of sports science research that indicate that "endurance" runners who are fast over 40m are the fastest over their chosen distance too. Sprinting – unlike slower running – does place more strain on your soft tissue (muscles, ligaments and tendons) and it is certainly the case that

unless you are a sprint athlete or already sprint regularly in your training, you will need to build up slowly before attempting to run flat out.

Sprinting uses your fast-twitch muscle fibres (see pages 77–8). These are the ones that, subject to relevant training, can increase muscle size and boost power, strength and speed. Runners who regularly run slowly will target primarily their slow twitch fibres (see page 75).

In chapter 3 we looked at drills related to the different parts of the running stride (see pages 27–35). These drills would be very much part of the sprint athlete's repertoire, the main difference being that they would usually be performed with greater speed. For instance,

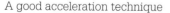

A good acceleration technique

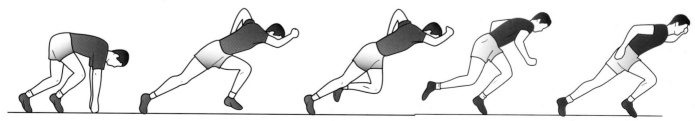

the leg cycling drill (exercise 3.6, page 31) could be performed at 100 per cent effort. Doing this will increase the potential of your body to "fire" its muscles quicker (where "fire" basically means triggering/recruiting fast limb and body movements). This mechanism can be trained in just the same way as endurance capacity – through repetition. The biggest difference is that the neural input has to be much greater (simply put, you need more mental focus). You can relatively easily slip into a 7–8 min per mile pace, for example, but to sprint 40m as fast as possible requires a totally different mental approach.

## Being "in the zone"

Fast twitch muscle fibre, or more specifically their motor units, are switched on one by one according to the "size principle". Basically, the more power/speed or strength that is required, the greater the need to fire the biggest and most powerful fast twitch motor units (motor units are bundles of muscle fibres and the nerves that switch them). To do this requires considerable neural energy. Your brain will send out electrical impulses to the muscles via the spinal cord and when these become powerful and rapid, so will your movements. To sprint you therefore need to be in the zone and mentally ready. You need to *want* to move fast. The running-specific warm-up (see chapter 4) can be very useful in this respect, particularly if the speed of the drills are gradually increased across sets and repetitions. You can also perform some specific exercises to boost your levels of arousal and ability to fire your fast twitch motor units (see panel below). This is useful if you're going to perform some fast intervals in training or are going to sprint.

When you are sprinting ensure that you have warmed up dynamically and have performed 3–5 40m runs which gradually increase in speed (known as "strides") before sprinting flat out. If you have not sprinted for a while, progress gradually and always underestimate what you think you can achieve. Recoveries should also be long, between 2–3 minutes between sprints for distances of 40m or less (sprinting over longer distances is more fatiguing and will require longer recoveries). As a rule of thumb you should not be out of breath when you sprint or perform sprint drills as fatigue will impair reactivity and good technique. Sprinting is a quality activity and as soon as your reactions begin to slow or you feel unable to move faster or maintain speed then you should take even more recovery or finish the session. In this instance, training slow will make you slow.

## Selected sprinting workouts

These workouts are best completed on a running track. As noted, you should be fully warmed up and recovered between efforts. Fatigue will impair performance. Relaxation is key to sprinting – tension will slow you down and is more likely to cause strain.

a) 6 x 60m sprints, from a standing start
b) 2 x 3 x 40m sprints from a standing start
c) 6 x 30m sprints with a 20m fast acceleration build-up
d) 20m accelerate/20m relax/20m flat out x 6
e) 4 x 80m sprints from a standing start

Take a full recovery between runs, i.e. 2–3 minutes. Where there are sets take 5–10 minutes between each set.

# Getting fired up to run fast

It is important that you are in the right frame of mind when you sprint or do faster track and road work, or hill sessions. As we have already seen, if you're not in the zone, you won't get the maximum benefits from your workouts. Sprinters often perform specific drills to "turn up" their neuromuscular system, so that they are in the right state of physical and, crucially, mental readiness to perform at 100 per cent speeds. Only a few repetitions (4–6) of these exercises should be performed prior to training sessions or competitions, where flat out or near-to-top running speeds are required. They should form part of the latter stage of your warm-up, when the body is "ready" for intense movements. Note: Many of the drills described in chapters 2 and 3 will serve a similar purpose, if performed at maximum or near to effort.

## Ex 6.1 Body rotation from short stance lunge position

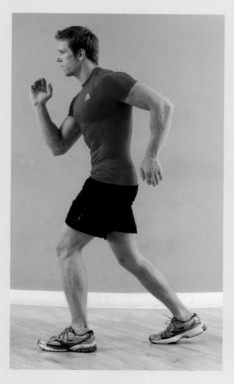 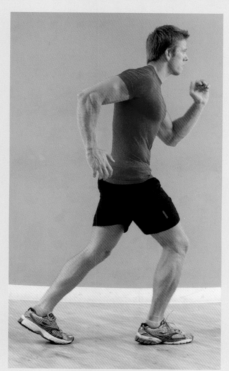

### How to perform

Take a medium step forward into a lunge. Keep your chest elevated and look straight ahead. When ready, turn as fast as possible through 180 degrees to reverse your stance. Initiate the movement by twisting through the ankles, knees and hips. Pause before rotating back the other way (do not do this in running spikes as your ability to turn will be restricted and there could be a danger of injury).

# Ex 6.2 Knee to hand drill

### How to perform

Assume a similar lunge position as for the exercise 6.1. Hold the palm of one hand out just above parallel to the ground. When ready, or to a command, drive the opposite leg to the hand as quickly as you can, so that your knee contacts your palm. Do not take your hand to your knee – the movement should be initiated from your hip flexor.

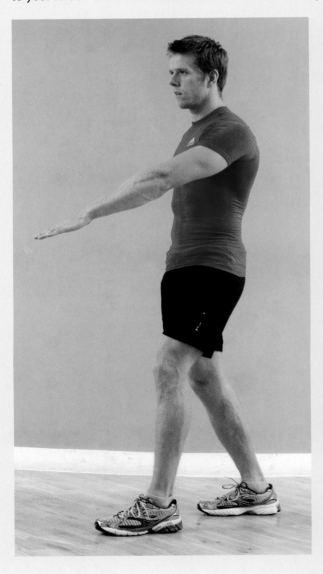
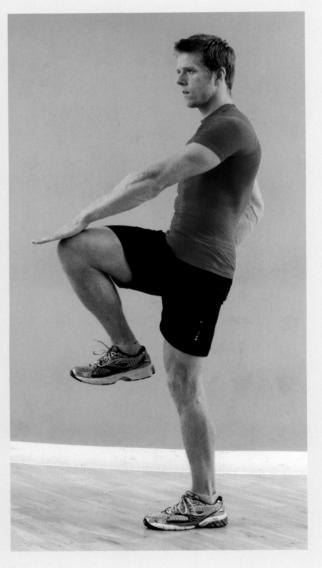

## Ex 6.3 Fast knees into sprint

### How to perform

On a running track (or other suitable surface), progress forwards by taking very small steps and lifting your knees to a near parallel-to-the-ground position. Build up your speed. Contact the ground on the balls of your feet and after about 10m start to lengthen your stride while trying to keep increasing your leg speed. Run on for another 20–30m. Progressing into running from the short, sharp knee lift movement will initially prove a challenge, but will enhance your ability to develop a faster cadence with practice.

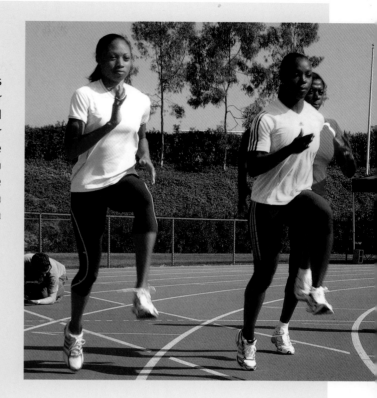

## Sprinting muscles

Sprinting (and running) requires a curvilinear action of the legs – study Usain Bolt's technique in slow motion, for example, and you'll see how his foot travels a curve from the drive phase, through recovery and into stance and foot strike. Although somewhat obvious, many runners and sportsmen and sportswomen perform too many drills, particularly high knees in an up and down way, which can lead to faulty run/sprint biomechanics.

### The hip flexors – the key sprinting muscle

Ask many coaches, runners and fitness trainers what they think are the most important muscles for running and they may well suggest that they are the quadriceps or the glutes; actually, it is the hip flexors. These muscles are crucial for a powerful and quick stride. They can be seen as the "pivotal" point (or rather muscle) of the running stride, "spinning" the legs below the hips and pulling them dynamically from rear to front over and over again. Conditioning these muscles appropriately will therefore have a direct impact on improving sprint and running speed, and many of the drills described in this book do just that (see chapters 3 and 4, for example).

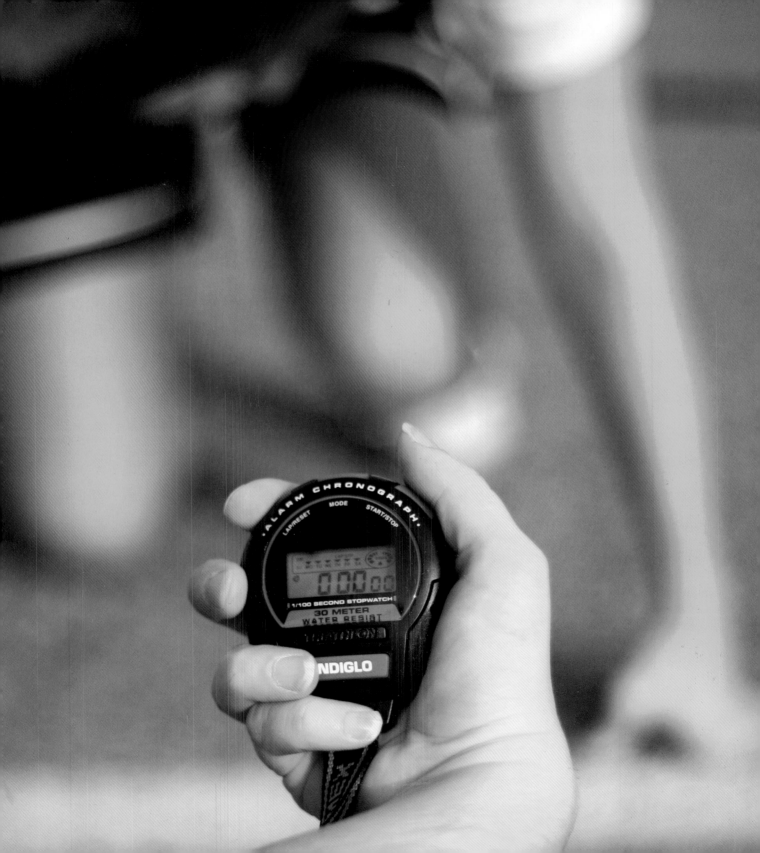

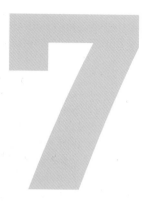

# planning your stronger running programme

Becoming a stronger runner rests heavily on the selection and implementation of the most appropriate conditioning ingredients at the right time. Just as you would meticulously plan your mileage it's just as important to plan in the same way the other aspects of your training. This chapter provides an introduction to training planning for stronger running. Its themes are followed up in the resistance training chapter (see chapter 8), which includes additional training plans and thoughts in particular on the development of maximum strength (see page 115) as a means to improve running performance.

Running coaches of elite/high level performers would not too long ago (and still do) send their athletes off to a weight lifting coach to learn the Olympic lifts (the "snatch" and the "clean and jerk") in order to develop "strength" for running. Although it does have its merits, such an approach often leads to the development of "strength for strength's sake" and not specific, usable strength for running. Today, specifically trained strength and conditioning coaches are relatively plentiful and this has certainly been beneficial to

runners in need of a relevant running-related conditioning training programme.

However, I believe it is vitally important for you as a runner or running coach to fully understand the process of how to structure a periodised (systematically phased) conditioning programme for running and to know what exercises and muscular actions to include. The conditioning components (mainly weights, circuits and plyometrics) must all be intertwined with the running parts. If you fail to view the whole process as a seamless one, you run the risk of a disjointed and less-than-performance-optimising running training programme. If you (or your coach) are in control, or you are at least properly managing the entire conditioning process, then it is more likely that you will establish a successful performance enhancing running programme.

## The training variables

The training variables are fundamental to constructing a progressive conditioning training plan – they inform and shape individual workouts and the overall plan. You will need to constantly reference these variables to produce the optimal running training plan for you. These include:

- Quantity
- Quality
- Duration
- Frequency,
- Intensity
- Load
- Rest

## Quantity

Quantity refers to the amount of training done, whether in a particular workout or as part of a particular training phase. It can be measured by the total weight lifted, repetitions or sets completed in the weights room or the number of ground contacts during a plyometric (jumping) session, for example.

## Quality

Quality usually reflects the intensity of a workout. For weight training, the amount of rest allowed between repetitions and sets and the speed of lifting reflect quality, for example. The longer the recovery, the greater the quality, as this will enable more powerful, more fade resistant (i.e. powerful) lifting to occur. The maximum strength method of weight training is a prime example of this (see chapter 8, page 115). A session with less quality could be a circuit resistance workout, which would usually only include light weights and also minimal

## The central nervous system (CNS)

The CNS is an important aspect – although often neglected one – of sports training. The CNS functions at both the conscious and unconscious levels and is crucial in terms of producing powerful and repeated muscular contractions in training and competition, as well as avoiding burn-out, reduced competitive and training performance and injury and illness. The CNS system sends nerve impulses to muscles, which are interpreted and acted on by the muscular system. The greater the magnitude and speed of these impulses and responses, the more forceful the contraction, with the result that you will be able to lift heavier loads and produce more power during weight lifting, for example. If this is then channelled appropriately through a relevant training plan, you will start to see an increased sports performance. Again, the strength of these impulses is reduced as you get tired, so as runner, if you want to increase your maximum strength, it is important to plan appropriately for rest and recovery so you get the most out of your training (see page 115, for more

information on why improving maximum strength can be important for the serious to elite runner in particular).

When strength endurance workouts (i.e. those that utilise high reps, a medium load and short recoveries) are performed, the CNS is taxed in a different way, although the outcome of fatigue is similar. If you do a lighter weights/body weight strength-endurance workout, then the speed at which you are able to complete your exercises will slow and fatigue of a more general kind will develop. More specifically, your movements will become less precise, slower and compromised by lactate and lactic acid build-up. Due to their intensity, the CNS will be weakened by these workouts. Again, it is therefore important that you factor in sufficient overall rest and recovery in your training plan. Failure to consider "CNS drain" can slow you in reaching your training objectives, and this is particularly true if you allow this to persist over time. It can also lead to over training and potential illness and injury (see box overleaf).

recoveries between each circuit exercise, so that the quality and precision of exercise performance is likely to fail due to the exerciser quickly becoming tired.

## Duration

This refers to the length of a training session on the more general level, or, on a much more focused level, to the lifting and lowering phases of a weights exercise or the time of hold of an isometric muscular action (when muscles work against each other to produce force, but no movement, such as pressing against a door-frame with your arms extended). The "speed of lift" of a weights exercise, like recovery, can also significantly affect training response in terms of hormone release and in terms of muscle fibre adaption (see page 73).

## Frequency

This refers to the number of times you train over a week, a month or other designated time span, or the number of times you perform a certain type of workout.

## Load

Specifically, load refers to the resistance that has to be overcome, i.e. the amount of load on a muscle. It is most applicable to weights sessions but also applies to vibration training (where the load is measured by the vibrational frequency and amplitude of the machine – see pages 151–2 for more information on vibration training). In this context, load refers to the magnitude of the training cycle. Microcycles (a period of training lasting usually a week to 10 days) should be progressed through light, medium and heavy load phases, so that the runner

adapts progressively (and safely) to the next level. Thus your running load would increase via an increase in weekly mileage/speed of runs/increased reps during an interval session and so on. If you don't factor in enough recovery time – within sessions and the overall training plan – you won't progress as well as you could.

## Rest

Rest is often neglected as a training variable, but it is just as important as the actual training you do. Training phases should include designated rest periods. Without them, you will not adapt optimally to the training because your body will fatigue more quickly. Rest can be seen to differ from recovery, in that rest involves non-training, whereas recovery involves specifically designated periods of stopping within a training session, i.e. between weights sets, for example, or intervals during a track workout.

# Macrocycles, mesocycles and microcycles

Macrocycles, mesocycles and microcycles are the terms used in training theory for different length periods of training.

## Macrocycles

The macrocycle is the overall training period. This is normally a year (although not necessarily a calendar year – some elite runners, for example, may work to a two-year cycle if they are preparing for a world championships). The macrocycle will also reflect the model of periodisation to be followed, i.e. one, two or even three peak (see page 79 for more detail).

## Mesocycles

Mesocycles are shorter periods of training lasting 4–6 weeks. They are structured against a specific theme – this could be for example, the development of anatomical adaptation (developing the necessary physical condition upon which to build more intense training) or maximum strength.

## Strength types

You can develop different types of strength in the weights room using varying combinations of reps, sets and loads. Load is normally measured in terms of weight lifted and is expressed as a percentage of one repetition maximum (1RM, see page 93 for how to calculate your own 1RM).

### Maximum strength

Maximum strength can be defined as the ability to overcome a very heavy resistance. In the weights room, this would involve lifting in excess of 85 per cent of 1RM and using very low reps and numbers of sets with long recoveries. Although you might not think so, these workouts are increasingly being seen as crucial in terms of athlete conditioning (for athletes in the widest sense), as they can increase your potential muscular horse-power when included within a specifically designed running conditioning programme. They form a key element of what is often known as the "maximum strength" method and can be of use to runners, especially those with elite aspirations (see chapter 8, page 115).

### Power

Power is traditionally trained in the weights room using loads in the region of 60–80 per cent of 1RM, over sets of 6–10 reps performed rapidly, but with control and with 1–2 minute recoveries between sets. Additional power-developing methods would include plyometrics and medicine ball throwing, for example. Both the former and the latter methods will generate faster and more powerful muscular contractions. Contemporary training theory has it that power (and therefore the ultimate, speed, jumping and throwing potential of the athlete) cannot be maximised without the athlete first gaining maximum strength, and then maintaining it. This can be achieved through a focused, targeted training plan (known as a periodised training plan).

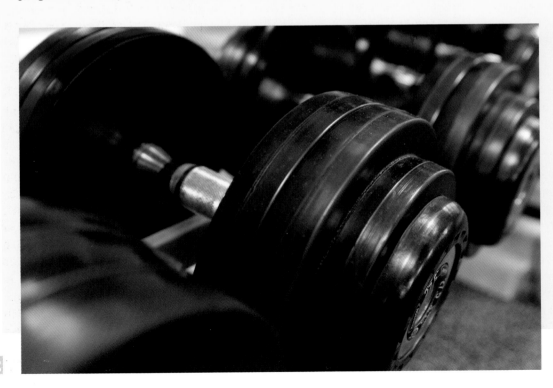

## Microcycles

Microcycles are the shortest training phases, lasting normally a week to 10 days. For the runner/coach these include all the specific session detail that would individually, but collectively, reflect the mesocycle's aims within the context of the macrocycle. So, this is where you would record in detail exactly what you are going to do in each of your training sessions.

## A power-endurance macrocycle training programme

Rowers are prime examples of athletes who need to sustain high power outputs over sustained periods of time – around 6 minutes in the case of their 2000m races. And, if you think about it, marathon runners need to do this too. Power-endurance development would traditionally comprise of circuit training and circuit resistance training methods (CRT utilises weights – see chapter 8, page 140). Both these types of training use high repetitions and short recoveries, with relatively light resistance. These workouts target your slow twitch and transitional (Type IIa) fast twitch muscles fibres (see pages 76–8). Transitional fibres when trained appropriately can become better suited to producing greater endurance or more power and speed.

Strength-endurance is another term that has been used to describe the ability of a muscle to "learn" to contract continuously when it gets tired, through relevant physiological adaptation. However, it is power-endurance that has greater relevance to improving your running as it embodies (and implies) quicker muscle contractions, which will speed up your running.

### Examples of power-endurance sessions

See page 93 for a detailed explanation of how to calculate your one repetition maximum (1RM).

- Low intensity: 4 x 20 reps at 50% 1RM
- Medium intensity: 5 x 30 reps at 60% 1RM
- High intensity: 6 x 15 reps at 70% 1RM

**Note:** intensity does not mean that certain sessions are superior to others, just that they have different effects on the body. However, it would also make sense for a runner new to this type of training to perform the low/medium intensity workouts initially as they build up relevant strength progressively.

**Note also:** You can alter the outcomes of these workouts (and all workouts) by applying the training variable (see page 70). For example, if you decided to increase the volume of the medium intensity session by adding more reps, for example, upping them to 50, then you would create a greater strength-endurance outcome. Conversely, if you were to reduce the number of reps to 20 and slightly increase the weight to 65 per cent 1RM, then, due to less fatigue, you would be able to generate more power. This workout would therefore have a better quality outcome overall.

## Understanding muscle fibre

We've talked about slow twitch and fast twitch muscles already in this book (see page 76), and it is important to understand how conditioning methods affect these fibres when it comes to optimising your running strength.

## Distribution of muscle fibre types

Most people are born with a relatively even distribution of fast twitch and slow twitch fibres – the range has been put somewhere between 45–55 per cent for both types. This tends to indicate that most of us are "made" and not "born" to a certain sporting predisposition. The exercise physiologists McKardle, Katch and Katch write, " .... studies with both humans and animals suggest a change in the biochemical-physiological properties of muscle fibres with a progressive transformation in fibre type with specific and chronic training."[1] In simple terms, you can change your muscle fibre type through training.

Table 7.1 displays the extent to which fibre type can be "altered" after training for selected endurance

# How muscles create force

Muscles pull on bones to create movement (or work against each other to create no movement, but still produce force), and they do this in numerous ways. As a runner, understanding how the different types of muscular action work will help you to get the most of your training plan.

### Concentric muscular action

A concentric muscular action occurs when a muscle shortens under load, as is the case during the lifting phase of a biceps curl (see figure 7.1a). It is the most common muscular action in sport.

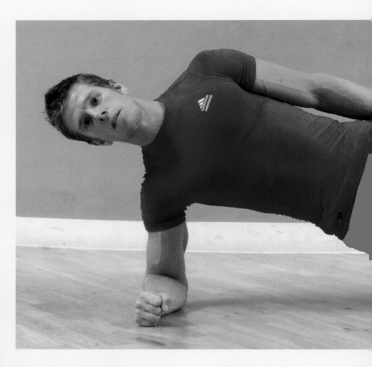

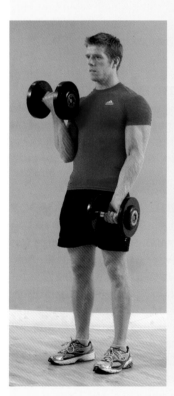
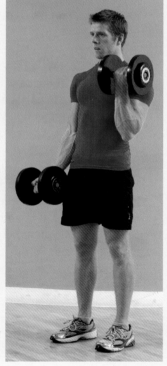

**Figure 7.1:** (a) The lifting phase of a biceps curl; (b) the lowering phase of a biceps curl.

### Eccentric muscular action

An eccentric muscular action occurs when a muscle lengthens under load, as is the case during the lowering phase of a biceps curl (see figure 7.1b). To give a running example, an eccentric muscular action occurs in the quadriceps when you are downhill running, as these muscles stretch to apply the brakes.

### Isotonic muscular action

Isotonic muscular action involves movement and the combination of concentric and eccentric muscular actions.

### Isometric muscular action

During an isometric muscular action, no movement occurs as opposing muscle groups work against each other or an object to generate force. Pressing against a door-frame is an everyday example which targets the chest and shoulders. Although not always hopping are typical plyometric drills. Plyometric training is also known as "elastic", involving the "stretch/shortening muscle cycle" and also the stretch reflex. Running is in itself a plyometric activity and you will be able to improve your stride and your speed even further by performing specific plyometric training workouts.

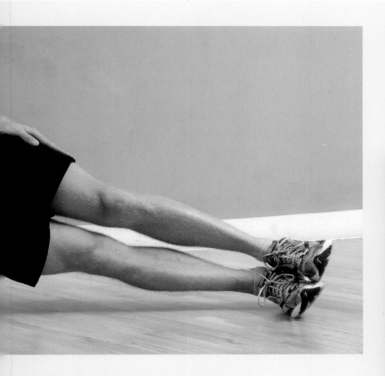

The plank generates an isometric action in the core muscles.

appreciated, isometric contractions are crucial to running and sports performance. This is particularly so for the core, as the back and abdominal muscles work in harmony to stabilise the trunk during sporting movement (see chapter 9 for a specific focus on core training for running).

## Plyometric muscular action

Plyometric muscular action involves the rapid transference between an eccentric and concentric action. The result is a very rapid and powerful release of energy, as the muscle/muscles stretch under load and then shorten powerfully. The action is akin to stretching out a spring (the eccentric action) and then releasing it (the concentric action). Bounding and

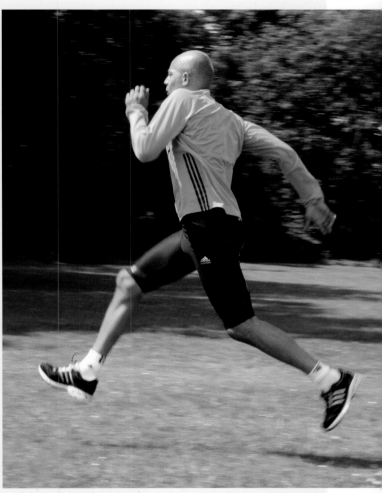

Bounding is a typical plyometric exercise, characterised by a rapid transference from an eccentric to a concentric muscular action.

**Table 7.1** Percentage of slow twitch fibre according to running distance

| Running distance/ sport | % of slow twitch fibre present |
|---|---|
| Sprinter | 15% |
| Average active person | 50% |
| Triathlete | 60% |
| Middle distance runner | 60% |
| Marathon runner | 80% |

activities. However, it is not so clear as to how long-lasting these changes are – of which more later.

## Muscle fibre types

Two basic muscle fibre types have been identified

- Slow twitch (type I, "red" fibres)
- Fast twitch (type II, "white" fibres). Type II fibres can be sub-divided into type IIa (intermediate) and type IIb variants (see page 77).

### Slow twitch muscle fibre

Slow twitch muscle fibre contracts almost half as fast as fast twitch fibre – 10–30 twitches per second, as opposed to 30–70 respectively. It has a good level of blood supply, which greatly assists its ability to generate aerobic energy, by allowing plentiful supplies of oxygen to the working muscles and numerous mitochondria. Mitochondria are cellular power plants; they function to turn food (primarily carbohydrates) into the energy required for muscular action, specifically adenosine triphosphate (ATP). ATP is found in all cells and is the body's universal energy donor. Whether your run is a fast anaerobic one or a steady lower pace one it is fuelled by the production of ATP and the actions of your fast and slow twitch muscle fibres.

Unlike fast twitch fibre, slow twitch fibre is much less likely to increase muscle size (known as "hypertrophy"). This is because slow twitch fibres are designed to produce aerobic energy and do not contain the cellular structure that fast twitch fibres do, which predisposes them to growth and more powerful anaerobic movements when subject to, for example, heavy resistance training. However, well-trained endurance athletes will have slow twitch fibres that are slightly enlarged, in comparison to sedentary individuals. The most noticeable training effects, however, are far less visible. Depending on the level of relevant endurance training, the unseen changes can include:

- an improved aerobic capacity caused by fibre adaptation, specifically an increase in mitochondria size, which increases the fibres' ability to generate aerobic energy;
- an increase in capillary density (the capillaries are the smallest of the body's blood vessels and are part of the circulatory system), which increases the ability of muscle fibre to transport oxygen and, therefore, increases the potential for greater energy; and
- an increase in the number of enzymes relevant to the Krebs cycle. The Krebs cycle is a chemical process that occurs within muscles – it permits the regeneration of ATP under aerobic conditions. The enzymes involved in this process can increase 2–3 times after a sustained period of endurance training.

*Lactic acid*

Blood lactate (or lactic acid) plays a crucial role in energy creation and not, as many people wrongly assume, only during the latter stages of intense exercise. In fact, blood lactate is actually involved in energy production at all times in our bodies.

The response to lactate generation is different according to muscle fibre type. If we look a little more closely, you will begin to see why the relationship between fast and slow twitch muscle fibre is crucial for optimum endurance.

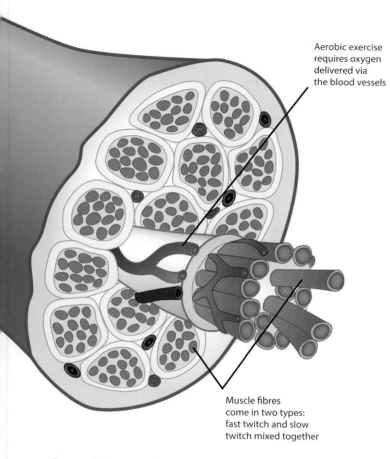

Aerobic exercise requires oxygen delivered via the blood vessels

Muscle fibres come in two types: fast twitch and slow twitch mixed together

Fast and slow twitch muscle fibres

Fast twitch fibres produce the enzyme lactate dehydrogenase (LDH), which converts pyruvic acid (PA) into lactic acid (LA). The LDH in slow twitch muscle fibre, however, favours the conversion of LA to PA. This means that the LA produced by the fast twitch muscle fibres can be oxidised by the slow twitch fibres in the same muscle to produce continuous muscular contractions.

When LA production reaches a level when it cannot be recycled to generate steady-state aerobic energy, endurance exercise moves into anaerobic territory, i.e. increasingly less reliance is placed on oxygen for energy production and more on stored phosphates. There will come a point under these conditions when the runner reaches their "lactate threshold", beyond which energy will be produced, depending on intensity and duration, increasingly anaerobically. At this point, further exercise becomes increasingly difficult and the runner will have to slow down and ultimately stop.

The well-trained endurance athlete is able to generate blood lactate levels 20–30 per cent higher than those of the untrained under similar conditions, which means that it takes longer for them to reach their lactate threshold. So don't just think that you need to train your slow twitch muscle fibres; training your fast twitch ones appropriately can very much improve your running performance.

### Fast twitch fibre and running

We've covered slow twitch fibre – so what about fast twitch fibre?

#### Type IIa

These intermediate fibres can, in elite endurance runners, become as effective at producing aerobic energy as the slow twitch fibres found in non-trained subjects. Like slow twitch fibres, Type IIa fibres (and their type IIb counterparts) will benefit from an increase in capillary density. In fact, it has been estimated that endurance training which recruits both fast and slow twitch muscle fibre can boost intra-muscular blood flow by 50–200 per cent.[2]

#### Type IIb

Research carried out[3] indicates that type IIb fibre can play a very significant role in sustained energy release to an extent greater than previously thought. Specifically, the researchers studied changes brought about through endurance training and specifically how muscular enzymes (enzymes are cellular catalysts that trigger chemical reaction within cells) were affected and concluded that type IIb fibres were equally important to endurance athletes in terms of their contribution to aerobic energy production as type IIa fibres.

Recent research indicates that intense training that targets both slow and fast twitch muscle fibre, such as fast track intervals with little recovery, can boost endurance ability specifically by boosting oxygen supply to working muscles by increasing the number of capillaries. In comparison, the adaptation that takes place in terms of an increase in aerobic enzymes is a much slower one via aerobic training methods. Consequentially, circuit resistance training and power-endurance training can be very useful conditioners for the runner.

### "Over slowing" fast twitch muscle fibre

Despite the fact that it is possible to train fast twitch fibre to take on more of a slow twitch blueprint through huge quantities of sustained aerobic work, taken to extremes, this may not actually be the best strategy for the endurance athlete.

The elite marathon runner Alberto Salazar – now coach to, among others, Mo Farah, the UK's finest ever distance runner – stated that he trained so aerobically hard in order to lose his ability to jump.[4] In other words, he was trying to covert all of his fast twitch fibres into slow twitch ones, in terms of their energy producing potential. He felt that if he could do this, then all his muscle fibres (now slow twitch predisposed) would be able to contribute all their energy to his focussed marathon running. However, for an endurance runner to lose all fast twitch speed and power ability is actually detrimental, and Salazar has now come to recognise this. For example, at the end of a closely fought marathon there may be a need for a sprint, which will require a fast twitch fibre input. Even more specifically there's the anaerobic/aerobic component of an endurance activity to consider and the speed needed to complete it competitively. An 800m race requires around 40 per cent anaerobic energy contribution and the runner must be fast and powerful to be successful – if they've neglected their speed through too much of an emphasis on steady-state aerobic work, then they will be off the pace. All things being equal, the greater your top speed the easier it will be to run at slower paces. Essentially, therefore, fast twitch fibre has to be trained appropriately to make for faster and more enduring running.

## Permanent or lasting? Training-induced changes to muscle fibre type

Despite virtually undisputed evidence that all muscle fibre types will adapt to a relevant training stimulus, it is less certain whether these changes will be permanent. One of the few studies to look more closely at the long-term effects of endurance training focussed on muscle fibre adaptation over a decade. Specifically, the study looked at the skeletal muscle from seven subjects, who had participated in ten years or more of high-intensity aerobic training, and six non-trained subjects, whose skeletal muscle was obtained through a muscle biopsy taken from the thigh muscle.

The results showed that the percentage of slow twitch fibres in the high-intensity aerobic training group was 70.9 per cent compared to 37.7 per cent in the non-training group. In terms of fast twitch fibres, the former group's average percentage was 25.3 per cent compared to 51.8 per cent in the non-training group. The researchers concluded that endurance training may promote a transition from type II to type I muscle fibre types and that this occurs at the expense of the type II fibre population.

However, despite this and other similar research, it seems that slow twitch (and fast twitch) muscle fibre tends to revert back to its pre-training status when you stop training (aging, however, may be an exception – see chapter 11).

## Muscle fibre has a fast twitch default setting

It seems to be the case that muscle fibre has a fast twitch default setting. The latter can be explained as follows: we use our slow twitch fibres much more than our fast twitch ones on a daily basis, so it would seem logical that a period of inactivity would de-train slow twitch fibre and allow fast twitch fibre to regenerate and convert back to a faster contraction speed.[5] The interesting and slightly less logical aspect of all this is the fact that this does not necessarily require speed training – research carried out on inactive muscle tissue, as a result of accident or illness (and even on dead bodies), has indicated an increase of fast twitch muscle fibre.[6]

## How to construct a year's periodised strength training running plan

We've already touched on the key considerations required to put together a periodised training plan, such as training variables, muscle fibre types and the role of the CNS. We now need to structure the conditioning plan – or the 'macrocycle'. Note: The considerations that follow do not specify running workouts, as this is not the aim of this book. Overviews of the types of conditioning workouts that are designed to fit into its various length phases (mesocycles and microcycles) are also provided (further examples, explanations and exercise descriptions can be found in chapter 8).

The example macrocycle provided shows how to periodise running strength within a year-long macrocycle. The sample plan is suitable for more serious runners, with 1–2 years of appropriate strength work behind them. Training maturity (see box on page 91) is a further important consideration, as a runner who is a) not physically mature and b) who does not have years of relevant preparatory conditioning behind them is unlikely to benefit from the plan and may not be strong enough to complete it (and therefore may put themselves at risk of injury). If you fall into this category, you should spend 6 months to a year building up relevant condition before attempting it – the strength-endurance and circuit workouts found on page 132 in chapter 8 would be a good place to start. Note: This plan includes lifting heavy weights and is based around the maximum strength method – a more detailed analysis of this method can be found in chapter 8, which also includes further ways to plan your running strength training development. These also have a more general application, being suited to the recreational runner.

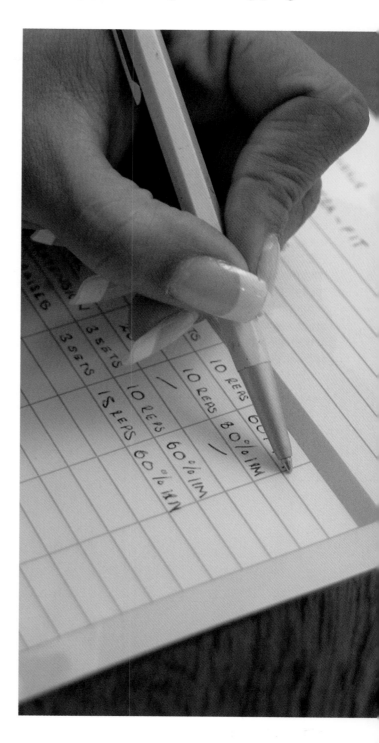

# Periodisation of running strength – an example 1-year macrocycle

Table 7.2 provides an example of a year-long strength conditioning macrocycle for a runner. Its various phases are colour coded and the diagonal lines represent the run over and declining/escalating training intensities of the phases as they merge into one another.

This example follows what is known as a "double periodisation" plan. Such a programme is designed to produce two peaks. For a runner, this could be for the later cross-country season/early spring road races and then a second peak in the summer months. This would suit a runner who has aspirations on the track or for summer 10k and 5k road races, for example. However, to reiterate, use this information with the right conditioning ingredients to create the relevant running programme for you. Note: The plan's phases could be lengthened and shortened to fit more closely to your specific plans.

Mesocycles are periods of training usually lasting 4-6 weeks. The content of these would be produced with a relatively broad brushstroke – the specific aims and objects and format of sessions (a "good overview") would be planned.

Microcyles are much shorter periods of training usually lasting a week to 10 days. The content of these would be produced with a much finer brush stroke, i.e. the actual specific content of individual sessions (reps, exercises, percentages of 1RM, where relevant for a weights workout) would be specified.

## Key to mesocycle colour coding
### Orange = preparatory
These mesocycles develop the specific and general condition required to handle the subsequently more intense and specific training load mesocycles. The emphasis would change from getting used to the exercises to be used in the following cycles to doing

**Table 7.2** Periodisation of strength for 1-year cacrocycle

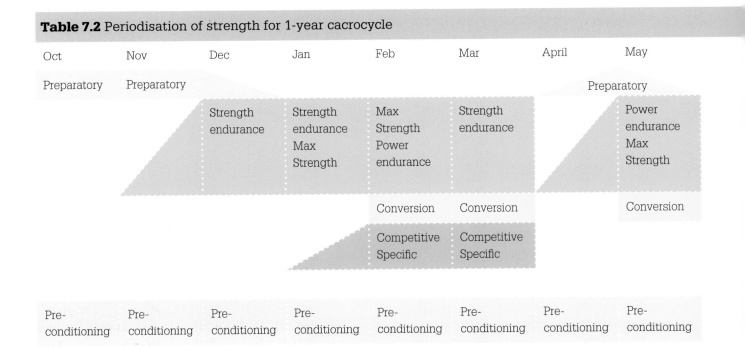

| | Oct | Nov | Dec | Jan | Feb | Mar | April | May |
|---|---|---|---|---|---|---|---|---|
| | Preparatory | Preparatory | | | | | | Preparatory |
| | | | Strength endurance | Strength endurance Max Strength | Max Strength Power endurance | Strength endurance | | Power endurance Max Strength |
| | | | | | Conversion | Conversion | | Conversion |
| | | | | | Competitive Specific | Competitive Specific | | |
| | Pre-conditioning | Pre-conditioning | Pre-conditioning | Pre-conditioning | Pre-conditioning | Pre-conditioning | Pre-conditioning | Pre-conditioning |

introductory, more specific strength-endurance sessions, for example. These sessions would have a greater emphasis on the development of slow twitch muscle fibre.

### Red = maximum strength/strength-endurance/power-endurance

These mesocycles develop fast twitch fibre and power endurance. They develop your ability to generate greater force, while increasing levels of fatigue tolerance.

### Yellow = conversion

These mesocycles progress the condition that has been developed in the strength-endurance/power-endurance/maximum strength phases and channel it more specifically into enhancing running performance. This is when plyometric exercises, for example, could have a greater role in the plan.

### Green = competitive

These mesocycles maintain the condition created in prior mesocycles and "hold" the runner in a continued state of competitive readiness. Particular attention must be paid to the state of the CNS and over-taxing it, which would be detrimental to performance (see page 70).

### Blue = transitional

This mesocycle is characterised by rest and recovery at the end of the training and competitive period and it is designed to restore the runner physically and mentally for the next training macrocycle.

### Light green = pre-conditioning

This is also referred to as pre-training (see chapter 1). This training runs throughout the macrocycle. It should be regarded as part and parcel of your conditioning and, although it should be emphasised mostly in the preparatory phases, it is crucial for specifically reducing injury potential throughout all other phases. A great example of a relevant exercise is the eccentric heel lower (calf raise) exercise (with or without weights on one or both legs), which can reduce the potential for an Achilles tendon strain when you emphasise the lowering (eccentric) action (see page 97). It is crucial for you and/or your coach to utilise the most relevant and "protective" pre-conditioning exercises, which reflect your individual running condition, injury and history.

As you can see from the macrocycle, the mesocycles overlap – this works to enhance transition between the phases and helps to optimise the channelling of your condition from phase to phase. Alongside this, the type of training used in each of the mesocycles complements or overlaps the previous one. For example, the single leg squat resistance exercise (see page 96) could be used throughout all the mesocycles, save for the transitional one, as it is a highly relevant conditioner, and all you would need to do to use the exercise at the relevant level is alter the load, volume and intensity, i.e. speed of movement, weight used as a percentage of 1RM and/or number of repetitions – in essence, alter

| June | July | Aug | Sep |
|---|---|---|---|
| Power Strength & Max Strength maintenance | Power Endurance & Max Strength maintenance | | |
| Conversion | Conversion | | |
| Competitive Specific | Competitive Specific | Competitive Specific | |
| | | | Transitional |
| Pre-conditioning | Pre-conditioning | Pre-conditioning | Pre-conditioning |

the variables according to the level you require (more on this later).

## What type of conditioning fits each mesocycle?

### Preparatory (orange)

These mesocycles are designed specifically to get you "ready to train". For a runner with a reasonable level of relevant running-specific conditioning behind them, the mesocycle (as indicated in the example) could last 2 months. However, for the more training-mature runner, 4 weeks may be all that is needed. For the less historically running-conditioned runner, perhaps slightly longer than 2 months will be needed. Circuit training, circuit resistance training, running drills and weights (with emphasis on really good technique) would all be staples of these mesocycles. In terms of the weight lifted, exercises would use loads between 50 and 75 per cent 1RM.

From the training variable load point of view, quantity is more important than quality. For example, a session of sprint drills (which are great specific running conditioning exercises – see chapters 3 and 4) could build up over a number of microcycles from 5 x 10 drills performed over 30m, with a walk back recovery and 2 minutes between sets of drills, to 20 x 10 drills performed on the same basis. Resistance exercises would similarly emphasise volume as the number of reps, sets and exercises would increase over the training period.

### Strength-endurance and maximum strength (red)

These conditioning phases are all about developing your ability to generate greater running power. More specifically by being able to optimally utilise your neuromuscular system, so that you can use as much of your power producing fast twitch muscle fibre as possible, as well as being able to tolerate increasing levels of fatigue, so you can run for longer. You should use isotonic, concentric, eccentric, isometric and plyometric muscular actions (see pages 74–5) in your conditioning programme in ways that will produce the best strength outcome for your running. In terms of weights exercises, you would aim to use loads in excess of 75 per cent 1RM.

### Conversion (yellow)

These phases take the maximum strength, strength-endurance and power and power-endurance generated by the maximum strength phase and transition it into enhanced running performance. Greater emphasis could be placed on plyometrics, for example, across these mesocycles, but remember to add these progressively – they should not be suddenly introduced, as this could lead to injury, which will reduce the effectiveness of the training programme. Maximum strength sessions would also continue to be "topped up" to maintain the previous gains that you have made. Quantity (as a training variable), however, would be progressively reduced, for example, in terms of fewer exercises being performed in a microcycle/workout to reduce fatigue, maintain freshness and permit peak competitive readiness.

### Competition (dark green)

In these mesocycles it is all about you getting ready to compete mentally and physically at your best. From a conditioning perspective, maximum strength training should again continue in order to reduce your chances of losing (or at least reducing) your ability to express maximum power. If this were to happen, then reduced competitive performance could result. One to two (much reduced in quantity) sessions could be scheduled, for example, into a 10-day microcycle and these should be kept well away from competitions (to avoid feeling tired on competitive outings) – it's crucial that the restoration of the CNS and the neuromuscular system takes place during this phase.

**Cycling is a cross-training and transitional phase option.**

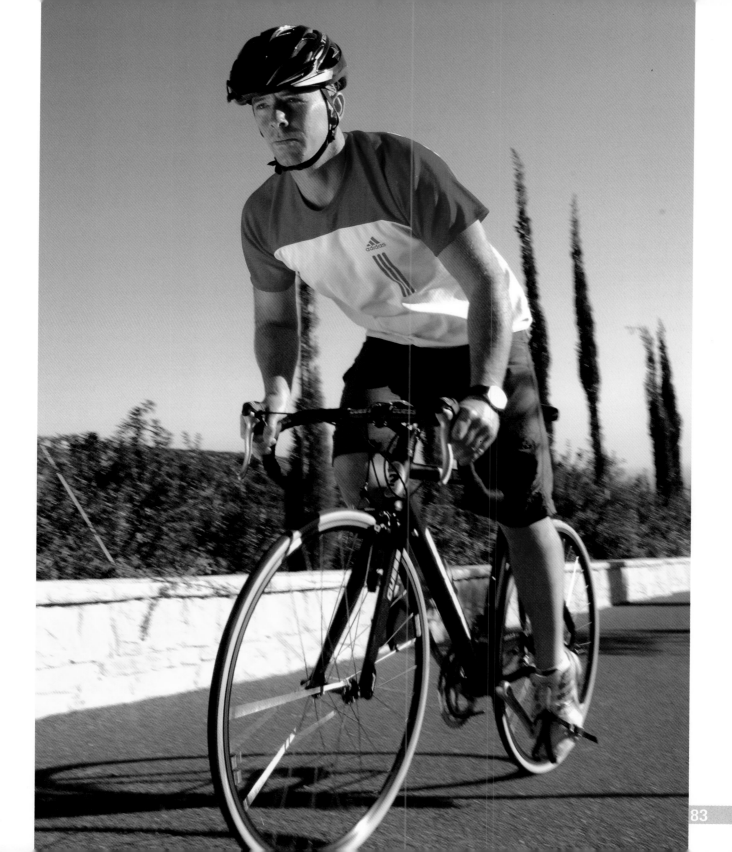

## Transitional (blue)

As indicated, this mesocycle occurs at the end of the training year. However, should an elite runner have a particularly tough indoor track or road or cross-country campaign, then a mini-transitional phase could be implemented in April as indicated on the sample plan. The emphasis should be on fun and on enjoyment of physical activity, so choose a physical activity that you enjoy, such as yoga, Pilates, walking, badminton or cycling. The key requirement is that fatigue should not be allowed to accumulate – you want to restore your physical, neural and mental energy. It's important to always monitor how you are feeling and responding to training and running (and other sources of stress) and adjust training levels accordingly.

## A note on cross-training

Cross-training – that's including other aerobic and anaerobic cardiovascular (CV) options such as swimming, pool sessions (wearing flotation jackets), cycling and rowing, can form a useful aspect of your training plan. The recreational runner and the elite runner alike can maintain CV condition and reduce the risk of overuse running injuries by incorporating such methods (see chapter 10 for more details).

## Pre-conditioning (light green)

As we have seen, this training should run in the background of all the other phases in the macrocycle and is designed to keep you injury free. Workouts within microcycles would specifically address this goal. Some of the exercises could be included within your warm-ups to save time. Exercises should be varied across the training cycle with new ones introduced progressively and the levels of fitness generated by previous ones topped up (see chapter 1 for a detailed focus).

## Phasing and transitioning between mesocycles

Below part of the macrocycle is highlighted to provide further clarity of understanding of the macrocycle planning process. We're looking specifically at the first 5 months of training for a plan starting in October.

In this example, on return to training in October after a transitional period, two months of preparation work follows. In November the start of the strength-endurance and maximum strength phases begins with a progressively increasing training load. Preparatory work would reduce quickly at the start of December.

Although it is not possible to show it on the diagram, you would not maximise the loadings in the November through to March (and beyond) in a purely linear fashion. Rather, to enable you to continuously adapt to the training loads, you should incorporate "light",

**Table 7.3** The first 5 months of a training macrocycle

| Oct | Nov | Dec | Jan | Feb |
|-----|-----|-----|-----|-----|
| Prepatory | Prepatory | | | |
| | | Strength endurance | Strength endurance Max Strength | Max Strength |
| | | | | Conversion |

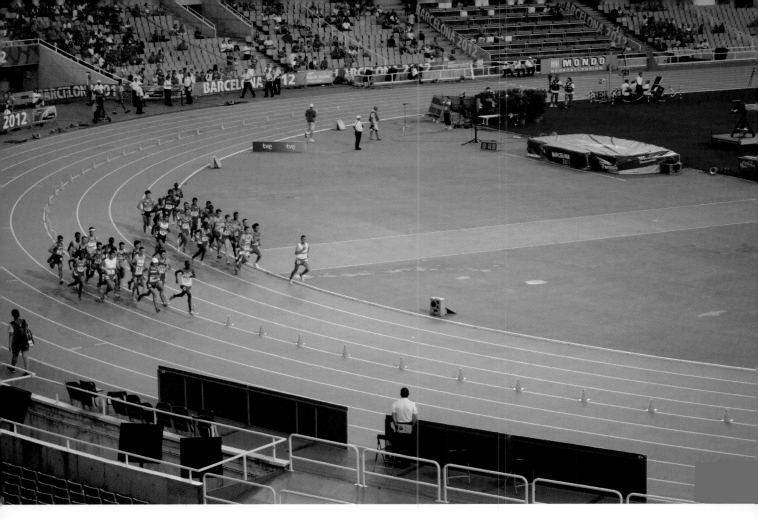

**Thorough planning will make for successful performances
– whatever your running level**

"easy" and "hard" microcyles. To control this, you and/ or your coach would need to apply the training variables to the conditioning and running session content. For example, the load lifted and the number of sets utilised during weight training could be manipulated – 4 x 8 reps at 85 per cent 1RM, on six exercises compared to 3 x 6 reps at the same load on three exercises. The former session is obviously harder than the latter, yet both develop maximum strength and power so quality would become ascendant over quantity.

## References

1   McArdle et al (1994), *Essentials of Exercise Physiology*, Williams and Wilkins
2   *Acta Physiologica Scandinavica*, 1984 Apr; 120(4): 505-515
3   *Journal of Applied Physics*, 1987(62):438-444
4   Salazaar – Nike lecture, Nike HQ Oregon, October 2002
5   *Journal of Sports Medicine and Physical Fitness*, 2000 Dec; 40(4):284-9
6   *Pflügers Archiv*, 2003 Mar; 445(6):734-40; E Pub 2003 Jan 14

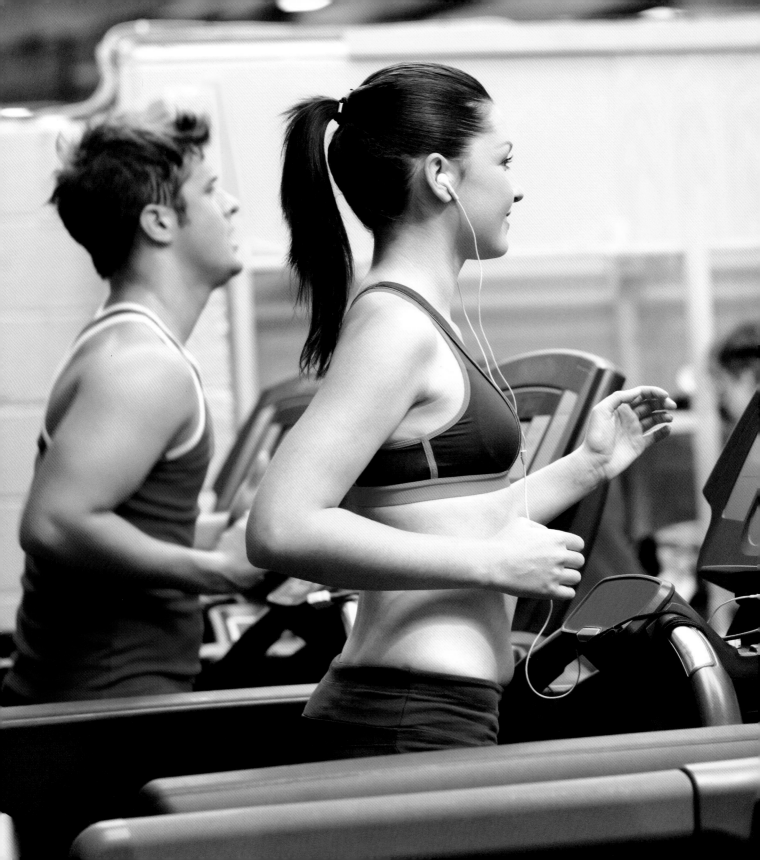

# resistance
# training

If you're a typical runner, it's more than likely that you're not a fan of weight training! Hopefully by now I've began to change your mind on that and on other forms of resistance training. Many runners neglect weight training, preferring to put in the miles on the road, track or in the countryside, rather than push out reps in the weights room. However, weight training – and other resistance training methods, such as circuit training and plyometrics (jumping-type exercises) – can be very beneficial to you. Some of these reasons have already been covered, for example, in terms of injury reduction (see chapter 1), so I've written this chapter to specifically outline the reasons why you should resistance train to boost your running speed and endurance.

The first section of this chapter deals specifically with weight training, the second with plyometric training and the third with body weight (circuit) training. We will also look at vibration training, which is becoming increasingly popular and is used for recovery and strength development purposes ever increasingly these days, as well as hill training. We also discuss how to include resistance training into your running training, so that you derive maximum benefits from it.

## Weight training and running

### Will weight training make you a better endurance runner?

To run for longer you need to improve the efficiency of your heart and lungs to pump greater quantities of oxygenated blood around your body. Over time your heart will improve its stroke volume and more blood will be supplied to the working muscles with decreased effort, i.e. lower heart rates. Consequently, your VO2max and your lactate threshold will improve (see page 77).

We have already seen how your muscle fibres adapt to training (see chapter 7, page 78). This adaptation occurs in response to cardiovascular (aerobic and anaerobic) training methods and resistance training methods. As I indicated in my introduction to this chapter, many runners are not great fans of weight training and until relatively recently this position has also been maintained by many sports scientists. There has been considerable debate within sports science and running circles as to the value of weight training for endurance performance (across all types of endurance sports, i.e. cross-country skiing, cycling and triathlon). We take a look at this debate in the next section.

Endurance training primarily targets slow twitch muscle fibres. These are known as, Type I or "red" fibres. You may also see/hear them called "slow-oxidative", which gives a big clue to their key energy producing function. These fibres are responsible for prolonged muscular action – they're the ones you want to rapidly reproduce if you are training for a marathon, for example. Steady state aerobic running will increase their numbers and their ability to process oxygen (oxygen is the fuel that ignites the chemical reactions within the muscle to produce constant aerobic power).

On the other hand, resistance training, including weight training and, in particular, medium- to heavy-load weight training, used in excess of 70 per cent of 1RM, targets fast twitch fibre. As we saw in chapter 7, there are two types of these "white" fibres: intermediate fast twitch ("Type IIa") and fast twitch ("Type IIb"). They are also known as "fast oxidative glycotic fibres", because of their ability to display, when subject to

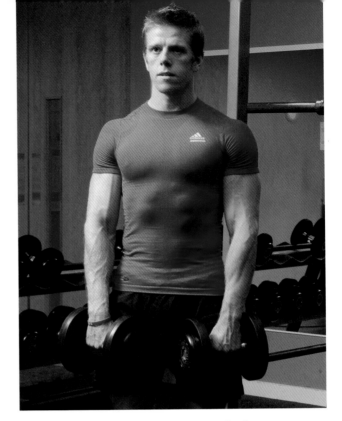
**Will weight training improve your running?**

the right training, a high capacity to contract under aerobic or anaerobic energy production, and "fast glycogenolytic fibres" as they rely solely on quick-start, high-powered anaerobic energy (Type IIa, Type IIb fibres respectively – see pages 76–8 for more detail on fibre types). Fast twitch muscle fibre is needed by sprinters and weight lifters for their "explosive" activities. A sprinter's foot may only be in contact with the ground for less than 0.09 of a second when flat out and yet in that time immense amounts of power will be produced.

Compared to slow twitch fibres, the "twitch rate" of fast twitch fibres is obviously much faster. In fact, fast twitch fibres have a twitch rate three times greater than slow twitch fibres – specifically 30–70 twitches per second. Consequently, some argue that training for strength and power using weight training and endurance methods at the same time can be counterproductive. Put simply, the potential to increase the power

## The interference effect

- Endurance training primarily targets slow twitch muscle fibres.
- Resistance training, including weight training, especially medium- to heavy-load weight training, used in excess of 70 per cent of 1RM, targets fast twitch fibre.

Many coaches and runners believe that the two forms of training cancel each other out, which has led them to avoid weight training altogether, as they attempt to get the best endurance out of their training. But recent research has indicated the opposite (see below).

producing capability of a muscle/muscle group and its motor units and impact on the neuromuscular system and the CNS through lifting weights is cancelled out by endurance training. This has been called the "interference effect" and has led to many coaches and runners eschewing weight training.

Prior to the turn of this century few research studies actually indicated that there was a direct benefit to weight training for the endurance runner (or endurance athlete in general) in terms of specific enhancement of endurance performance. However, more recent research has begun to indicate that the maximum strength method (see chapter 7, page 72) can have positive outcomes. The secondary benefits of weight training are much less disputable, i.e. assisting with injury prevention. Weight training and other resistance exercises (see chapter 2) can also increase co-ordination and balance, making for more efficient running.

## Weight training and endurance training – the interference effect

This section looks in more detail at the arguments for and against weight training for running and more general endurance activity.

### Rowing and weight training

Let's start by taking a look at another endurance sport – rowing. Rowing taxes both the aerobic and the anaerobic energy systems to the max. It's estimated that the aerobic contribution is 70% and the anaerobic 30% when rowing 200m – the Olympic race event. On completion the rower will be totally exhausted, if they have committed 100%. Researchers looked at the effects of three different weight training programmes on 18 varsity rowers during their winter training.[1] One group performed 18–22 high-velocity, low-resistance repetitions, while another did low-velocity, high-resistance repetitions (6–8 reps). All exercises were rowing-specific and were performed on variable-resistance hydraulic equipment four times a week for five weeks. A third group did no resistance training.

### Equipment options

As a runner you may not be a member of a gym and/or have access to a substantial amount of weight training equipment. As such, I've designed many of the workouts that follow so that they can be performed using easily obtainable kit. In fact, you could do many of the workouts at home. Relevant items of kit include Swiss balls, Powerbags and dumbbells. However, some workouts do require that you use heavier resistances, as well as fixed weight machines – both of which would be found in a typical gym. These later workouts are designed to develop the "strength types" – maximum strength and power in particular – and for the runner with elite-level aspirations, who will need to follow the maximum strength methodology (see page 115).

All groups carried out their normal endurance rowing training. When tested on a rowing machine, the researchers discovered no differences between any of the groups in terms of peak power output or peak lactate levels. So it appeared that weight training had no benefit in terms of increased endurance. Similar findings were made by researchers at the University of Ohio,[2] whose elite male weight-training rowers displayed no increase in VO2max, when compared to a rowing only group, who improved their VO2max by up to 16% per cent during pre-season training.

### Swimming and weight training

Moving to a different sport – swimming. Researchers looked at the effects of resistance training on 24 experienced swimmers.[3] They were surveyed over 14 weeks of their competitive season. The swimmers were divided into two groups of 12 and matched for stroke specialties and performance. One group resistance trained three days a week, on alternate days for eight weeks, the other group did no weight training. Weights

89

were selected for their swimming specificity – both fixed and free weights were used, i.e. it would make sense that if an exercise shared a similar movement pattern to those used in swimming, then there would be greater transferability. The swimmers performed three sets of 8–12 repetitions of lat pull downs, elbow extensions, bent arm flyes, dips and chin-ups. The weights were progressively increased over the duration of the training period, so it's likely they were performing relatively powerful contractions that would target fast and slow twitch fibre.

Two weeks away from their major competition a tapering period took place (tapering results in a reduced training load so that the athlete comes to a peak physically and mentally in readiness for competition). So what was the result of this piece of research? As with the rowing studies, it was found that weight training did not directly improve swim performance, despite the fact that those swimmers who combined resistance and swim training increased their strength by 25–35 per cent.

### Cross-country skiing and weight training

Researchers from Finland considered the effects of weight training and other power training methods on the performance of cross-country skiers – long considered the epitome of aerobic athletes.[4] Seven skiers performed explosive strength training, as well as plyometrics. In the weights room they performed 80 per cent of 1RM squats regularly, moving into maximum strength territory. Another eight of their peers performed three weeks of endurance based, high-repetition strength training for the legs and arms. At the end of the survey no difference in VO2max or the aerobic or anaerobic threshold was discovered.

With all this research from various sports it does seem that, in terms of a specific contribution to the markers of improved endurance performance, weights and other resistance methods have no, if any, effects.

However, let's look a little more closely. Perhaps there are some mitigating and explanatory circum-

stances. In the swimming research, weight training was introduced into the competitive phase of the swimmers – perhaps not the best time to do so. It's possible that the swimmers' performances could have actually been impaired by the added training load, rather than improved by it, with the extra and unfamiliar training load increasing fatigue levels. The fact that their performance levels remained the same is not, therefore, as bad as it first sounds. And the skiers? The researchers got one group of skiers to perform very dynamic exercises and admitted that their ability to express peak power did improve accordingly, but perhaps this was not optimally (if at all) channelled into improved potential performance, by following a long-term relevantly constructed training programme (we saw how to develop such a strategy in chapter 7).

The sports scientist Saziorski[5] suggests that, as theirs was an ultra-endurance sport, perhaps weight training held little direct relevance to improving their performance in the first place – he believes that maximum strength is of little importance to sports with a maximum strength requirement of less than 30 per cent. However, this position has been challenged by other elite sports conditioning experts, such as Tudor Bompa (see maximum strength method page 115), and further research into the benefits of maximum strength training.

The rowing findings are more difficult to deal with, but there is a possible answer. It's argued that when an endurance athlete reaches a certain level of performance strength – this can be developed through their everyday CV training or with weight training (or other resistance training) – that further improvements in weights-produced strength will not deliver further improvements in their sports performance. As the rowers in the studies were all at a high level, it could be argued that this explained the outcome, as they already had more than enough "performance" strength developed over years and years of correctly executed rowing technique.

Research from Canada offer a very succinct explanation as to why weight training and endurance training may not work together.

"Some of the most important and influential factors that result from physical conditioning occur at the cellular level in the muscles, that is, the majority of training effects are peripheral. The number and size of mitochondria (cellular power plants), the amount of myoglobin (iron and protein binding protein found in muscle tissue), the amounts of ATP and CP (adenosine triphosphate and creatine phosphate – energy producing chemicals) that are stored and the concentrations of key enzymes associated with particular energy systems are increased. Training is specific and selective of the types of muscle fibres used. That selectivity will determine the nature of training effects and the type of performance that is improved."[6]

Basically, this research argues that training different energy systems at the same time can produce a confused physiological affect. For example, how can fast twitch type IIb fibre be expected to gain in size and power-generating capacity through weight training if it is being relentlessly bombarded in the same training phase by extensive, slow distance work or intense interval training? After all, this is training that, as well as bolstering its slow twitch counterparts' aerobic efficiency, also causes Type IIa (and Type IIb) fast twitch fibre to become more enduring.

All this would seemingly throw into question the benefit to be had from weights (and other resistance training methods) to the endurance athlete. However, it seems that the key for the runner (and all other similar endurance athletes) in terms of generating performance benefits from weight training is the construction of a relevant training programme and the most appropriate

## Running level, training maturity and response to resistance training

When you start a training programme for the first time, positive adaption is almost guaranteed. A novice runner who starts weight training can expect to see positive returns on their running. However, a "serious" training mature runner (one who has perhaps been training for five or so more years consistently and who enters annual marathons) is perhaps less likely to gain such a positive transference into their actual running performance. Their mind and their muscles and their training regularity will be somewhat set and "new" training methods will require longer to take hold (they'll also be more likely to be affected by the "interference effect" – see page 88). However, as indicated in this section and other chapters of this book, there are coaches and runners and a mounting number of research findings that do back up the merits of resistance training as a means to improve endurance running, crucially if you follow the "right" programmes (the benefits of resistance training and in particular the use of heavy weights for sprinting is virtually undisputed).

use of exercises and reps, sets and loads. The level of your running and your "training maturity" also need to be factored into the equation (see box above). You also need to very carefully consider the training variables (see pages 69–71) when combining endurance and CV training. Maximise your recovery time between the two methods in your workout schedules and perhaps even consider weight training your legs in a separate specific workout, or even a mesocycle. The latter option will give you greater strength to apply to your running by being developed away from a heavy running endurance training phase.

## The importance of rest and session spacing

Researchers looked at the effects of weight training on aerobic/anaerobic CV performance.[7] Sixteen male collegiate athletes experienced in strength training, sub-maximal aerobic training and high-intensity anaerobic interval training, took part in a research study to see if the type and intensity of aerobic training affected concurrent strength training after four, eight and twenty-four hours of recovery. One group performed steady state work at 70 per cent of maximum heart rate (MHR) and another 95–100 per cent intensity intervals with 40 per cent MHR recoveries. Both groups then performed 1RM strength testing on the bench press and leg press.

Not surprisingly, it was discovered that for both the steady state and the interval training groups strength training gains were compromised by the endurance work unless adequate rest was allowed. Specifically the participants' leg muscles were negatively affected by their aerobic training, as measured by the leg press, although bench press performance was perhaps more obviously not affected. Consequently, the researchers recommended that at least eight hours be allowed between aerobic training and strength training if both workouts were to be performed on the same day and that lower body strength training should be performed on a different day to any aerobic training.

Expanding this planning theme further, you could consider the possible benefits of developing strength in a specific training cycle away from your endurance training, particularly at the beginning of the training year to gain the most from it. This can reduce the potential of the interference effect and provide you with the best conditions to develop stronger, fatigue-resistant muscles. The focus on one form of training will allow for unfettered physiological adaptation. Periodic returns to weight and other resistance training microcycles could then be used to "top-up" strength levels.

Under these conditions, a Canadian study of rowers[8] discovered that a group that strength trained for five weeks, before five weeks of endurance training, profited from a 16 per cent increase in VO2max and a 27 per cent improvement in lactate tolerance after the 10-week programme, while a group that trained in the reverse order only gained a 7 per cent increase in VO2max and displayed no improvements in lactate tolerance. The explanation? It's likely that the "strength before endurance" group gained quality rowing muscle without physiological compromise and were able to use it to row harder and faster with greater fatigue resistance when they endurance trained. Working out for weight training gains alone, may have enabled them to push beyond their "normal" previously conditioned rowing power levels (this reflects the "maximum strength" method of improving endurance performance with weights – see page 115).

Getting your resistance training to compliment and approve your running will require careful planning and account for many of the factors we have seen in this section. See pages 93–5 for more information on how to ensure that you, as a runner, get the best from your weight training.

### Avoiding overuse injuries

Runners are a tenacious bunch and run for the somewhat obvious reason that they want to run! If and when an injury prevents running, there can be a significant psychological impact. Varying training by incorporating resistance training and cross-training (see chapter 10) can reduce the chances of injury and can also stimulate the runner both mentally and physically. Getting a structured training plan together that factors in all these ingredients is crucial in this respect (note: the information provided in chapter 7 as well as that in this chapter, will be useful in helping you to create the right training programme for you).

# Weight training workouts for runners

In this section I provide a selection of specific running weight training workouts. These are particularly suited to the recreational runner (runners of elite standard, or with elite aspirations, and also sprinters should see pages 116–17 for ways to train with weights to develop maximum strength as a running enhancer). **Note:** In reference to the information provided in chapter 7 regarding strength types, the following workouts develop strength and power endurance.

The workouts should be performed during specific mesocycles. One such cycle could be at the start of your training period/year, where three sessions could be performed a week for 4–6 weeks, with these reduced to one to two sessions thereafter, for maintenance purposes during subsequent mesocycles as your running quantities and intensities increase.

As indicated, the workouts focus on strength and power endurance development rather than maximum strength, i.e. the weight lifted (where relevant) is not greater than 60 per cent of your 1RM. Most runners should be able to lift these weights safely, although if you have no previous weight training experience, then do spend time building up your strength levels and learning correct exercise technique.

## One repetition maximums (1RMs)

The workouts that follow indicate the weight you should lift (where applicable) as a percentage of one repetition maximum. This is the maximum amount of weight you could lift on any one exercise, i.e. once, and provides the loading for the exercises in the workouts. For example, if your 1RM squat was 100kg (i.e. when you perform a squat, you can do it with a maximum load of 100kg), 70 per cent of your 1RM would be 70kg and 50 per cent, 50kg and so on.

If you are new to weight training, then it is not advisable to go for 1RM tests, nor in many cases even for the experienced weight trainer is this necessary. You can use fatigue and the inability to complete a further repetition/repetition during a set/sets with good form as a guide.

### Formula for calculating 1RM
The information below offers a further way of calculating a notional 1RM.

- Reps x weight x 0.0333 + weight
- So, if you manage 6 reps at 70kg, 6 x 70 = 420 x 0.0333 = 13.98 + 70 = 83.98kg estimated 1RM

**Table 8.1** Using good form as a guide to weight training

| Percentage (%) of 1RM | No. of reps possible before good form goes |
|---|---|
| <90 at 1RM | 1–3 |
| 80–90% | 3–8 |
| 70–80% | 8–12 |
| 60–70% | 10–16 |
| 50–60% | 12–20+ |

**Note:** You should see the above as a guideline only as, dependent on your fitness, the exercise and your specific weight training history, you may be able to complete more or less repetitions. This is particularly the case with weights below 70 per cent of 1RM where prior endurance training and mental perseverance can often result in higher numbers of reps being performed.

## Core exercises

**Note:** Core exercises are provided in the workouts to spread the load placed across the body during each weights session – although most emphasise the leg muscles. The importance of the core for running and many more core exercises are provided in chapter 9.

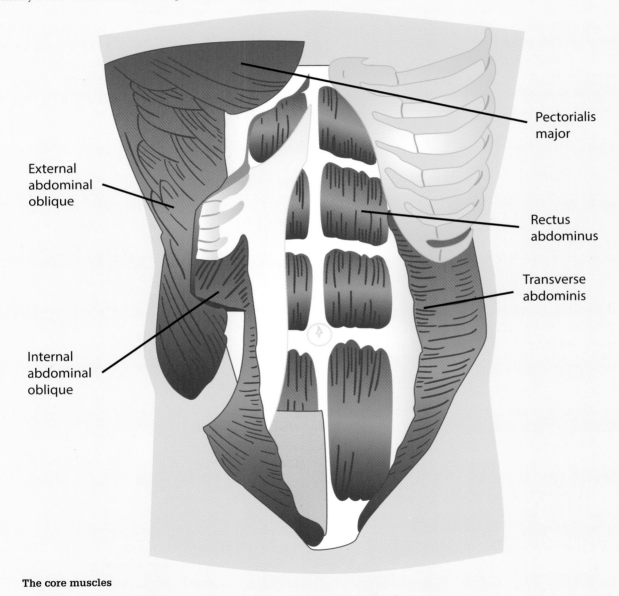

External abdominal oblique

Internal abdominal oblique

Pectorialis major

Rectus abdominus

Transverse abdominis

**The core muscles**

These workouts target slow and intermediate fast twitch muscle fibres making them more complimentary to an aerobic emphasis, steady-state mileage training programme. Doing this will also minimise the interference effect (see page 88). Aim to perform these workouts on the days when you are not running. These sessions will also enhance your running robustness, i.e. reduce the potential for injury.

## Weight training workout 1

### Purpose
This workout will specifically strengthen your running muscles, develop strength and power endurance and reduce the potential of injury.

### Suitable for
All runners

### Weight to lift
A medium-heavy weight (60 per cent of 1RM), where applicable.

### How to progress the workout
Increase the number of reps gradually to 20 (20 on each leg, where appropriate) and then the number of sets to six, again progressively – doing this will add to the strength-endurance aspect of the workout. Although a 30-second recovery is indicated, depending on your fitness and the progression of the circuit you may wish to increase or decrease this. Perform a set of each exercise and then another and so on with a designated recovery, before returning to repeat a set of each exercise – the workout is being performed in a circuit format.

### Warming up for weight training sessions
Warm up with a couple of minutes of jogging and then perform some functional movements for all body parts, such as arms swings and marching on the spot. Then do a set of the weights exercise at a moderate weight before progressing to the loadings specified.

### Weight training workout 1

| Exercise no. | Exercise name | Reps | Sets | Recovery |
|---|---|---|---|---|
| Ex 8.1 | Single leg squat | 10 (each leg) | 3–6 | 30 sec between legs and after sets are completed |
| Ex 8.2 | Single leg dead-lift | 10 (each leg) | 3–6 | As above |
| Ex 8.3 | Walking lunge with twist | 10 (each leg) | 3–6 | 30 sec between reps and sets |
| Ex 8.4 | Calf raises | 10 (each leg) | 3–6 | As above |
| Ex 8.5 | Swiss ball hamstring curl | 10 | 3–6 | As above |
| Ex 8.6 | One leg dynamic bridge | 10 (each leg) | 3–6 | 30 sec between legs and after sets are completed |
| Ex 8.7 | Swiss ball roll-outs | 10 | 3–6 | 30 sec |

# Exercise descriptions

## Ex 8.1 Single leg squat

**Targets**
This exercise targets calf muscles, quads and glutes and will promote balance and ankle, knee and hip strength.

**How to perform**
Hold the dumbbells at arm's length. Stand on one leg and tuck the heel of the other up towards your bottom. Bend your standing leg to lower your body. Keep your knee over your ankle and focus on dropping your bottom straight down over your heel. Push back up and extend your hips as you do so. Try to keep your torso upright, maintaining the natural curves of your spine and look straight ahead.

**Training tips**
Gripping the floor by squeezing your toes can assist balance – you may find it easier to do this exercise barefoot.

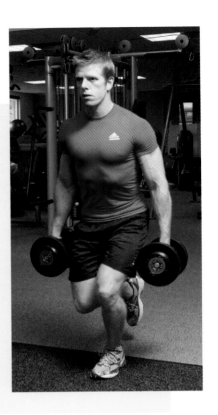

## Ex 8.2 Single leg dead-lift

**Targets**
This exercise targets the hamstrings, glutes and lower back.

**How to perform**
Hold dumbbells at arm's length by your sides. Stand on one leg and maintain a slight bend at the knee. Tuck the heel of your other leg up towards your bottom. Lean forward from your hips, while maintaining the natural curves of your back. Lower the dumbbells to just in front of the standing foot. Next, pull back up to the start position by engaging your hamstrings, glutes and lower back.

**Training tip**
Do not squat the weight up – emphasise the movement of your hips and lower back.

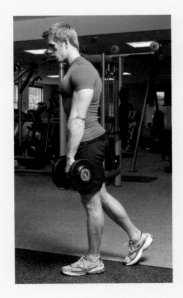

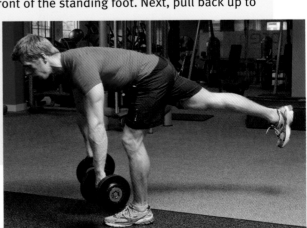

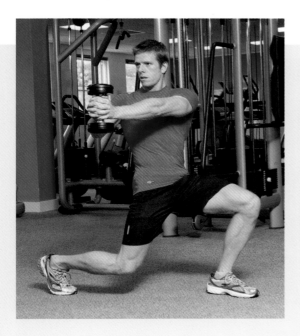

## Ex 8.3 Walking lunge with twist

### Targets
This exercise targets the legs, glutes and torso and will also improve balance.

### How to perform
Hold the weight (medicine ball/dumbbell/kettlebell) at arm's length in both hands and parallel to the floor. Take a large step forward into a lunge and twist in both directions and then back to centre, before stepping forwards into another lunge.

### Training tip
This exercise is not suited to using a heavy weight.

## Ex 8.4 Calf raises

### Targets
This exercise targets the calf muscles – notably the larger, more powerful gastrocnemius.

### How to perform
Support the weight across your shoulders if using a barbell, or hold dumbbells at arm's length. The exercise can also be performed on a calf raise machine. Rise up onto your toes. Lower under control. Keep looking straight ahead, maintaining the natural curves of your spine.

### Training tip
Emphasising the lowering phase of the movement (the eccentric muscle contraction), by using a five count, will develop eccentric strength in the Achilles tendons and other supporting soft tissue structures of the lower leg, reducing potential injury risk (see chapter 1, page 2 for more detail). Use a step riser to increase the range of movement of the exercise, but only work within a comfortable range of movement for you.

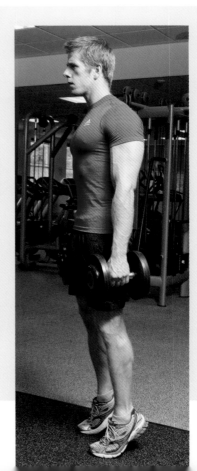

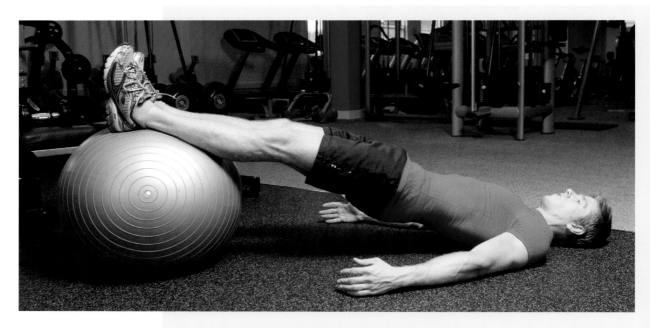

## Ex 8.5 Swiss ball hamstring curl

### Targets
This exercise targets the hamstrings and glutes and will also build core strength.

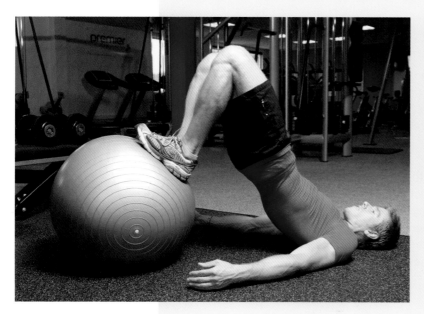

### How to perform
Place your heels on the Swiss ball and lift your hips, keeping your back and head on the ground. Position your hands by your sides (your weight should be supported through your upper back). Keep your hips high and glutes contracted as you pull the ball in and then roll it away. Work slowly with control.

### Progression
Perform one leg at a time.

## Ex 8.6 One leg dynamic bridge

### Targets
This exercise targets the hamstrings and glutes.

### How to perform
Lie on your back and place your hands in line with your shoulder. Lift your hips and squeeze your glutes. As you do this, lift one leg to a near parallel/parallel-to-the-ground position. Lower under control and repeat with the other leg.

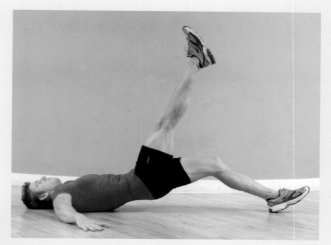

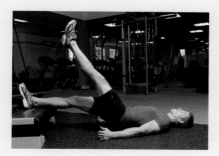

### Variation
The exercise can also be performed with the working leg supported on a bench (see photo).

## Ex 8.7 Swiss ball roll-outs

### Targets
This exercise targets the core – the deep stabiliser muscles of your trunk are essential for controlling the twisting and turning forces that are generated when running – this exercise dynamically targets them.

### How to perform
Kneel and place your hands to the sides of a Swiss ball (position a mat/towel under your knees for cushioning). Lean into the ball, maintaining a neutral spine and extend your arms and body to roll the ball away. Next draw the ball back in and repeat. Contract your abdominal muscles strongly throughout.

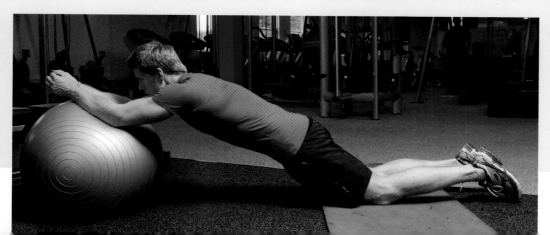

# Weight training workout 2

## Purpose
As workout 1 (see page 95)

## Suitable for
As workout 1

## Weight to lift
A medium-heavy weight (60 per cent of 1RM), where applicable.

## How to progress this workout
Increase the number of repetitions by 2–5 on a week-by-week basis up until you complete 40 reps (or 40 on each leg where appropriate). You can increase sets systematically – don't significantly increase reps and sets at the same time. You can also reduce recovery systematically until you take just 5 seconds between sets and exercises.

To make the workout even more demanding instead of performing circuit style, perform "in-series". To do this you will need to perform all sets of the exercise to be performed first before moving on to the next (different) exercise. So you would perform 20 lunges to the left and to the right, pause for, for example, 20 seconds and then complete another set. You would only move onto the next (different) exercise once you completed all your sets of the first exercise. In-series workouts are more demanding than circuit-style ones.

| Weight training workout 2 | | | | |
|---|---|---|---|---|
| **Exercise no.** | **Exercise name** | **Reps** | **Sets** | **Recovery** |
| Ex 8.8 | Lunge | 20 (each leg) | 3–6 | 20 sec after sets are completed (complete all reps on one leg and then on other) |
| Ex 8.9 | Single leg calf raise | 10 (each leg) | 3–6 | As above |
| Ex 8.10 | Squat | 20 (each leg) | 3–6 | 20 sec between sets |
| Ex 8.11 | Alternate knee to elbow crunch | 20 | 3–6 | As above |
| Ex 8.12 | Swiss ball squat with hold | 20 | 3–6 | As above |
| Ex 8.13 | Sprint arm action with dumbbells | 40 (left and right movement equals 1 rep) | 3–6 | As above |
| Ex 8.14 | Lateral lunge | 20 (each leg) | 3–6 | 20 sec after sets are completed (complete all reps to one side and then on other) |

# Exercise descriptions

## Ex 8.8 Lunge

### Targets
This exercise targets the legs and glutes.

### How to perform
Stand with your feet shoulder-width apart. Hold dumbbells at arm's length or support a barbell/ Powerbag across your shoulders. Take a large a step forward into a lunge, bending both legs to a 90-degree angle. Keeping your front foot flat on the floor, push back through your heel to the start position. Pause and repeat. Repeat all reps on one leg before changing to the other.

### Training tips
Keep the knee of your front leg over its ankle throughout the exercise (do not let the knee or your toes press forward – to reduce potential knee strain).

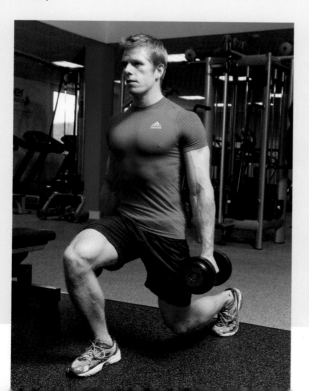

## Ex 8.9 Single leg calf raise

### Targets
This exercise targets the calf muscles. As with the double calf raise variant (see workout 1, exercise 8.4), this is a great exercise for strengthening the Achilles tendons so that they are more injury resilient.

### How to perform
Hold dumbbells at arm's length or support a barbell/Power bag across your shoulders. Stand with your heels preferably over a low step. Lift the heel of one leg a couple of centimetres from the floor. Extend the ankle of your other foot to lift your body. Pause and lower under control. Complete all your reps on one leg and then swap legs.

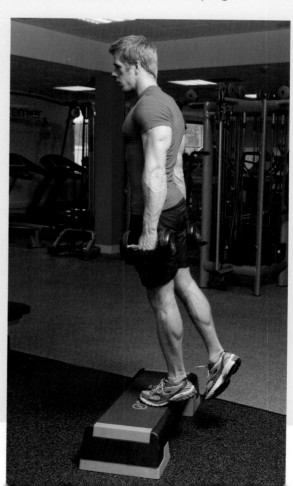

## Ex 8.10 Squat

**Targets**
This exercise targets the quads, hips and glutes.

**How to perform**
Stand with your feet hip-width apart. Position a barbell/
Powerbag across the back of your shoulders or hold dumbbells
at arm's length. Look straight ahead and lower your thighs to a
parallel or near parallel-to-the-ground position. Keep your heels
on the ground and maintain the natural curves of your spine.
Push back up through your heels to return to the start position.

**Training tips**
Do not allow your knees to rotate inwards or outwards.

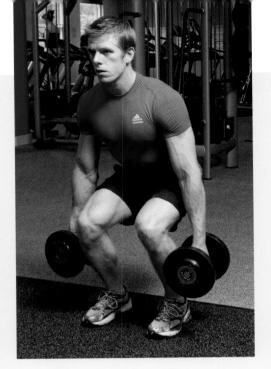

## Ex 8.11 Alternate knee to elbow crunch ("chinnies")

**Targets**
This exercise targets the core and hip flexors.

**How to perform**
Lie on your back and then fold at the middle as you bring one shoulder to its opposite knee.
Return to the start position and repeat with the other knee and shoulder. Keep your hands
by your ears and elbows out throughout the exercise. Don't let your upper back or legs
touch the ground during each set. Maintain a steady and fast, but controlled, pace.

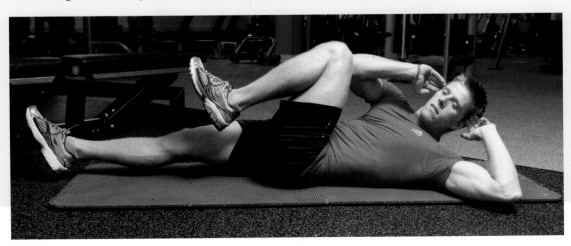

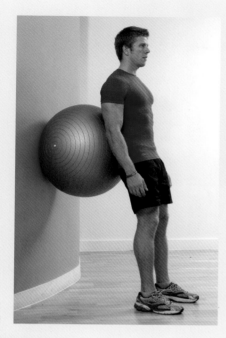

## Ex 8.12 Swiss ball squat with hold

### Targets
This exercise targets the legs, glutes and core and involves an isometric contraction as well as concentric and eccentric ones.

### How to perform
Place a Swiss ball in the small of your back and against a wall. Position your feet shoulder-width apart. Brace your body and bend your legs to squat so that your thighs are parallel or near to the ground. Hold for a count of five and then push back up through your heels.

### Progression
Perform one leg at a time, by extending the non-squatting leg to the front and holding it off of the ground. Varying the muscular actions in a workout and an exercise will prove more taxing on the body (the hold employs an isometric action).

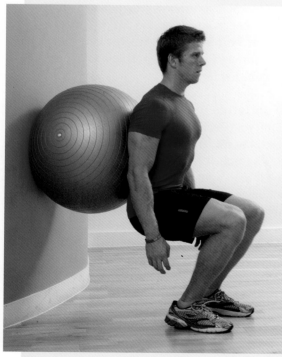

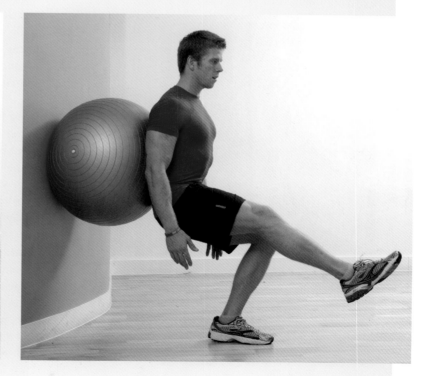

## Ex 8.13 Sprint arm action with dumbbells

### Targets
This exercise targets the arms, shoulders and core.

### How to perform
Take a large step forwards into a lunge. Hold dumbbells in your hands and bend both arms so that there is approximately a 90-degree angle at your elbows. Brace your core and pump your arms backwards and forwards as if sprinting. Keep your chest elevated and look straight ahead. Try to remain relaxed as you complete your sets.

### Tip
Keep your shoulders down and relaxed and use light dumbbells for this exercise (of 2–5kg).

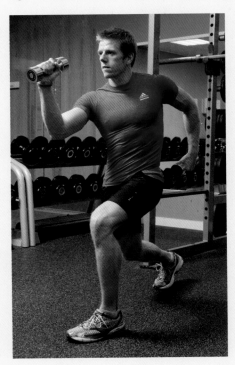

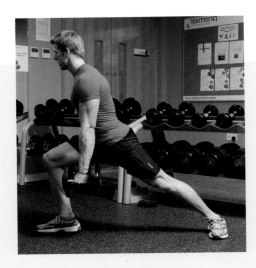

## Ex 8.14 Lateral lunge

### Targets
This exercise targets the legs and glutes. The lateral movement will improve your balance as well as leg strength – lunging sideways brings in to play numerous small muscles that will have to work to stop you falling/losing balance. This will transfer into improved running by allowing your ankle and knees in particular to cope with lateral forces, which are, for example, created by running on uneven surfaces (for further examples of such exercises see chapter 1).

### How to perform
Stand with your feet shoulder-width apart. Hold dumbbells at arm's length by your sides or place a barbell/Powerbag across your shoulders. Take a large step to your right, to about a 15-degree angle. Turn your ankle as you do so, so that your toes are in alignment with your knees. Doing this will ensure the safe hinging of your knee joint. Lower your front thigh to a parallel/near parallel-to-the-ground position. Keep your knee over your ankle as with the standard lunge – think "dropping bottom to heel". Push back though your heel to the start position. Complete all your reps to the right and then to the left. You can co-ordinate your arms with your legs or place your hands on your hips.

# Power developing workouts

The following two workouts are designed to develop greater power, rather than endurance.

## Weight training workout 3

### Purpose

To specifically strengthen the muscles used in running, develop strength and increased running power, and reduce the potential for injury. This workout requires access to a gym with a leg press, leg curl and leg extension machine and low pulley/seated row machine and has a specific preconditioning function (see chapter 1).

**Note:** "How to perform" descriptions may vary due to differing equipment design. If you are unsure as to how to use an item, seek advice from a qualified instructor.

### Suitable for

All runners with a background of lifting heavier weights

### Weight to lift

A medium-heavy weight around 75 per cent 1RM.

### About this workout

As indicated this workout has more of a power aspect to it then workouts 1 and 2, as the weights are heavier (75 per cent of 1RM). Movements must be powerful but controlled. Try lifting to a one count and lowering to a two count, where applicable. Exercises such as the leg curl and the leg extension, which target the quadriceps and the hamstrings respectively, are less relevant to the biomechanics of running, but are very useful for reducing injury to the knees and hamstrings respectively. The low pulley seated row exercise targets the shoulders in a way that's similar to the running movement, albeit bilaterally as opposed to the unilateral running arm movement. The inclusion of the jump squat adds to the dynamic nature of the workout – use a lighter load for this exercise, around 30 per cent 1RM. If you have not performed this exercise before, do so with just body weight for a couple of weeks before adding load. To reduce potential strain on the back, hold dumbbells at arm's length.

Core exercises have also been included to balance the demands placed on the body.

Take 1 minute's rest between sets and 2 minutes between sets, and perform the exercises in-series. If you need more recovery, extend your recovery periods – you want to be able to perform the repetitions crisply and with power. If you begin to struggle, reduce the load, number of sets or truncate the session.

| Weight training workout 3 | | | | |
|---|---|---|---|---|
| **Exercise no.** | **Exercise name** | **Reps** | **Sets** | **Recovery** |
| Ex 8.15 | Leg extension | 10 | 4 | 60 sec between exercises |
| Ex 8.16 | Leg curl | 10 | 4 | 60 sec between exercises |
| Ex 8.17 | Seated row | 12 | 4 | 60 sec between exercises |
| Ex 8.18 | Leg press | 10 | 4 | 60 sec between exercises |
| Ex 8.19 | Plank | 30 sec hold | 4 | 60 sec between exercises |
| Ex 8.20 | Calf extension on leg press machine | 16 | 4 | 60 sec between exercises |
| Ex 8.21 | Jump squat | 6–8 | 4 | 60 sec between exercises |

## Ex 8.15 Leg extension

### How to perform

Place the tops of your feet under the machine's pads and your hands by your sides. Sit upright or with a slight backward lean (if the machine has a backrest). Extend your legs to lift the weight, keeping your thighs in contact with the bench. Don't swing the weights up – "squeeze" out each rep. Control the movement back down to ensure you develop eccentric strength in your quadriceps.

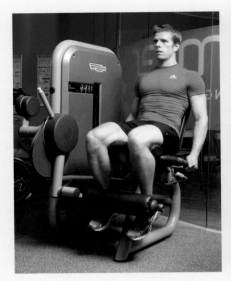
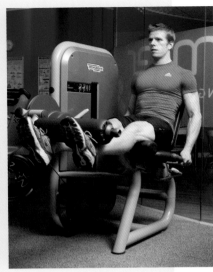

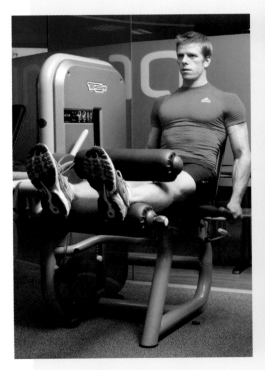
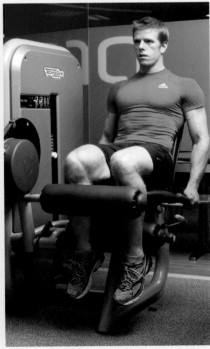

## Ex 8.16 Leg curl

### Targets

This exercise targets the hamstrings.

### How to perform

Sit on the machine and place the back of your ankles over the machine's pads. Position the lap pad just above your knees. Hold onto the grips on the lap pad (or place hands by your sides depending on the design of the machine). Pull the weights in towards you and then extend your legs to return to the start position. Keep your back against the seat throughout.

## Ex 8.17 Seated row

### Targets
This exercise targets the upper back, shoulders and core (forearms).

### How to perform
This exercise can be performed on a specific seated row machine or using a low pulley machine. Place your feet against the machine's foot rests, grasp the grips (straight bar or triangle attachment). Sit up, maintaining a slight bend at your knees. Pull your elbows back, keeping your forearms parallel to the ground. Brace your torso throughout. Aim to pull the bar/grips into your upper abdomen. Return the weights to the start position under control. Do not let yourself be pulled towards the weights.

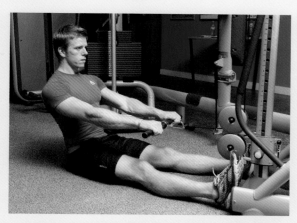

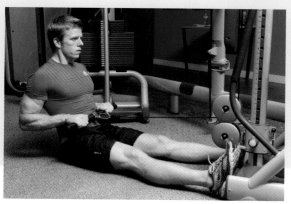

## Ex 8.18 Leg press

### Targets
This exercise targets the glutes, quadriceps and hamstrings.

### How to perform
Adjust the seat so that you legs are able to fully extend. Place your feet hip-width apart on the plate. Grasp the handles by your sides and press the weights away from you keeping your feet fully on the plate. Do not allow your knees to splay outwards as you push. Control the return of the weights.

### Variation
Perform one leg at a time.

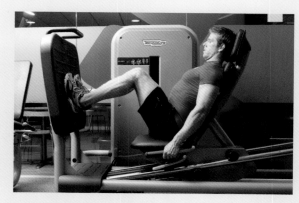

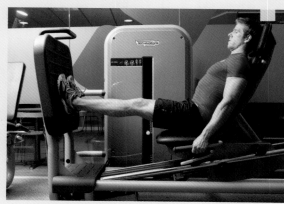

## Ex 8.19 Plank

### Targets
This exercise targets the core using an isometric contraction.

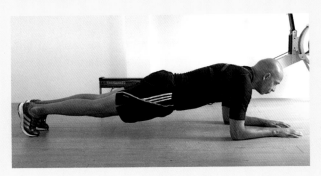

### How to perform
Assume a prone position, with your elbows next to your head and your forearms extended in front of you. Lift your body from the floor using your legs and arms and brace your core. Maintain a straight line through the back of your head, shoulders, bottom and heels. Hold for the designated duration and lower under control.

### Training tips
Remember to breathe throughout the exercise. Have a training partner place a broomstick across your back, head and shoulders so that you can attain the alignment required of the exercise if necessary. Many people perform the exercise without proper form and in doing so use the "wrong" muscles, which risks injury.

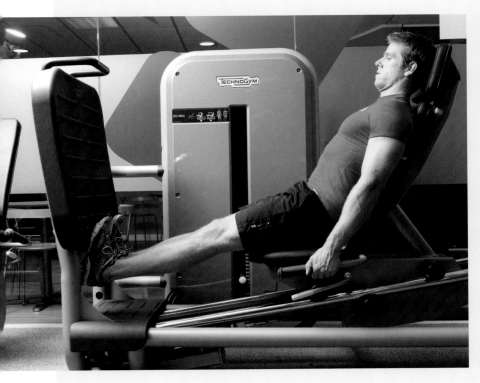

## Ex 8.20 Calf extension on leg press machine

### Targets
This exercise targets the calf muscles.

### How to perform
Assume the same starting position as for Ex 8.18, the leg press. With legs extended, press the plate further away from you using just your ankles. Control the weights on their way back and repeat.

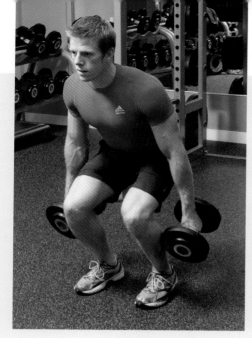

# Ex 8.21 Jump squat

### Targets
This exercise targets the hamstrings, quadriceps, glutes and calf muscles plyometrically.

### How to perform
Place a barbell/Powerbag across your shoulders and pull it firmly down, or hold dumbbells at arm's length by your sides (those new to this exercise should just use body weight and then progress gradually to using dumbbells). Stand with your feet hip-width apart. Bend your knees to a three-quarter squat position, then dynamically extend your ankle, knees and hips to jump into the air. Land on the balls of your feet, set yourself and repeat.

### Training tips
Try to put as much energy as you can into each jump – don't go through the motions. Doing this will supply neural energy to your fast twitch muscle fibres and in particular their larger motor units. This will produce greater power that, with regular performance, can boost your running.

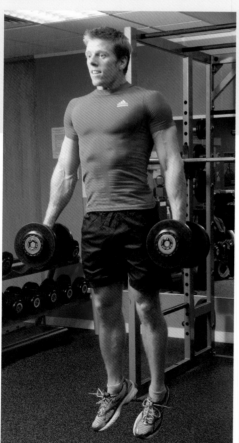

## Power combination training
Combining weights and plyometric exercises into a workout is known as "power combination training". These workouts have been shown to enhance the power output of your fast twitch muscle fibres through a process known as "potentiation". It's as if one form of training primes the other (or more specifically your muscle fibres) for a greater power expression. By including the jump squat in workout 3, we incorporated some power combination training into that workout.

# Weight training workout 4

## Purpose
To specifically strengthen the muscles used in running, employing on occasions running-related movements, such as the step-up drive. It will also develop overall running-related strength, power and robustness.

## Suitable for
All runners, with a suitable background in lifting heavier weights

## Weight to lift
A medium heavy weight around 80 per cent 1RM where applicable, or unless otherwise stated.

## About this workout
Like workout 3, this workout has more of a power aspect to it using weights set this time at 80 per cent of 1RM. Movements must be dynamic but controlled. Try lifting to a one count and lowering to a two count, where applicable.

If you need more recovery, extend your recovery periods – you want to perform the repetitions crisply and with power. If you begin to struggle, reduce the load, number of sets or truncate the session.

| Weight training workout 4 | | | | |
|---|---|---|---|---|
| **Exercise no.** | **Exercise name** | **Reps** | **Sets** | **Recovery** |
| Ex 8.22 | Step-up drive | 6 | 4 | 60 sec between legs and after sets |
| Ex 8.23 | Up right row – dumbbell | 8 | 4 | 60 sec between sets |
| Ex 8.24 | Split squat | 8 | 4 | 60 sec between legs and after sets |
| Ex 8.25 | High pulley woodchop | 6 | 4 | 60 sec between left and right sides and after sets |
| Ex 8.26 | Farmer's walk on tip-toes (perform with 50% of 1RM) | 20 sec | 4 | 60 sec between left and right sides and after sets |
| Ex 8.27 | Prone row | 10 (5 on each side) | 4 | 60 sec between left and right sides and after sets |

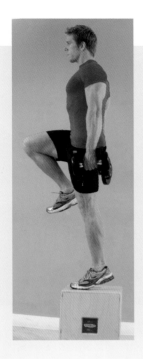

# Ex 8.22 Step-up drive

**Targets**

This exercise targets the hip flexors, quadriceps, core, glutes and calf muscles and is also a great exercise for developing a powerful running hip action and leg drive.

**How to perform**

Stand in front of a sturdy exercise bench or use a step aerobics riser. Hold dumbbells at arm's length by your sides. You can also use a barbell or Powerbag placed across the back of your shoulders. If using the former, have a training partner on hand to help position the bag on your shoulders, and for the latter, use squat racks. Powerfully step up onto the bench, driving your other thigh up at the same time so that it reaches a position parallel to the ground. Rise up onto your tip-toes as you do so. Keep your torso braced, upright and look straight ahead. Place the extended thigh's foot back onto the bench and step back down, leading with your stepping leg. Complete all your repetitions on one side and as described before changing legs.

# Ex 8.23 Upright row (dumbbell variant)

**Targets**

This exercise targets the upper back, rear shoulders, biceps and core. The main relevance of this exercise to the runner is in developing torso strength. Most weights exercises target more muscles than those that are actually moving – specifically your core muscles which need to be fully engaged when performing this exercise.

**How to perform**

Stand with your feet just beyond shoulder-width apart. Hold dumbbells in each hand at waist-height, with your knuckles facing forwards and dumbbells parallel to the floor. Pull both the dumbbells up symmetrically so that they reach a position in line with your sternum. Your upper arms should be parallel to the floor. Lower with control and repeat. Keep your torso braced and look straight ahead at all times.

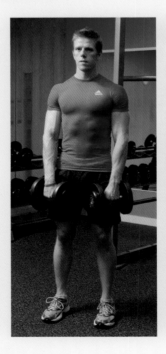
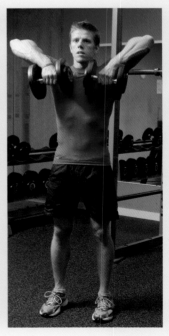

## Ex 8.24 Split squat

### Targets
This exercise targets the quadriceps, glutes and hamstrings and balance and requires strength through your torso, balance, which all makes for a great exercise for runners.

### How to perform
Place a barbell or Powerbag across the back of your shoulders. You can also hold dumbbells at arm's length by your sides. If using the former, have a training partner on hand to help position the bag on your shoulders, and for the latter, use squat racks. The exercise can also be performed by straddling a bar and holding it at arm's length. Take a large step forward into a lunge. This is the start position. Bend your front knee to lower your body. Your front knee should not pass in front of your toes and

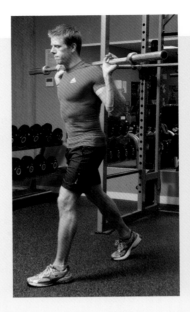
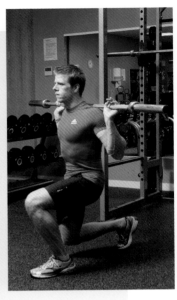

your rear leg should not touch the ground. Keep your trunk upright and look straight ahead. Extend your front leg to return to the start position.

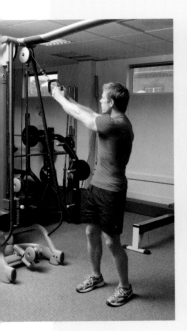
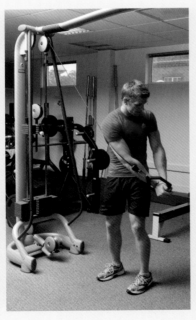

## Ex 8.25 High pulley woodchop

### Targets
This exercise targets the shoulders, chest and parts of the upper back and torso. Performing this exercise will strengthen the muscles that rotate and control the rotation of your trunk, which will help you to develop a trunk that is better able to withstand rotational forces (as well as generate them).

### How to perform
Stand side on to a high pulley machine with your feet just beyond shoulder-width apart. Take hold of the cable grip in both hands over your shoulder. Pull the grip down and across your body towards your opposite hip, rotating your body as you do so. Return the weights to the start position with control. Complete your set and repeat to the other side.

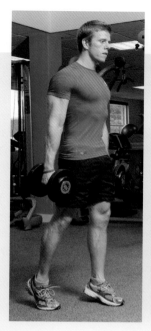
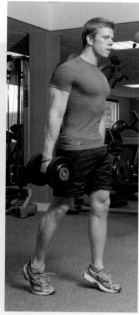

# Ex 8.26 Farmer's walk on tip-toes

### Targets
This exercise targets the legs, arms, core. It will also hit your calf muscles as they have to hold your body in position as you walk up and down. This is a great exercise for strengthening your lower legs and Achilles tendons and will help combat injury.

### How to perform
This unusual exercise requires you to grasp dumbbells at arm's length by your sides and lift up onto tip-toes and walk in a straight line, taking small steps. Turn and then walk back to the start position. Continue to do so for 20 seconds. Try to keep the dumbbells relatively still.

# Ex 8.27 Prone row

### Targets
This exercise targets the upper back and shoulders.

### How to perform
Set an incline bench to a 45-degree angle. Lie on the bench with the dumbbells at arm's length and your knees resting on the "seat" part of the bench. Leading with your elbows, pull your arms back. Pause at the top of the movement for a second and then lower the weights slowly and with control to the start position.

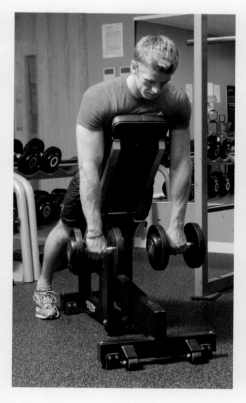
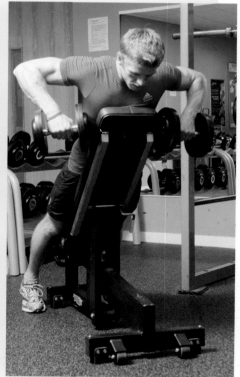

## Why train with heavy weights?

As we've seen in this section and in chapter 7, there are advocates and research studies that indicate that heavy weight training – using loads in excess of 80 per cent of 1RM – can boost running performance, whatever your distance. However, these workouts require technical proficiency in terms of being able to perform the exercises without risk of injury and, obviously, a solid base of prior weight training experience and considerable willpower to to be able to tackle them. The positioning of these types of workouts within the training programme is also crucial.

In chapter 7 we looked at an example of a double periodisation conditioning plan that displayed how to fit these sessions into a progressive strength training for running plan. However, it's also possible to use another type of macrocycle with maximum strength sessions performed at the start of the training year, when mileages are relatively low. In that case, muscle fibre won't be challenged significantly by "two types" of training at the same time (see "interference effect", page 88), while fast twitch fibres in particular will be given every opportunity to adapt optimally. This approach requires you as the runner to be experienced in lifting heavy loads and, despite the emphasis in early mescoycles, progress to these loadings must be made over at least a 4-week preliminary period of training. Such an approach would produce stronger, more powerful muscles, which will allow you to add endurance later.

As the macrocycle progresses and training emphasis changes then this ability may gradually decrease; to keep it topped-up you could incorporate carefully

**Why train with heavier weights?**

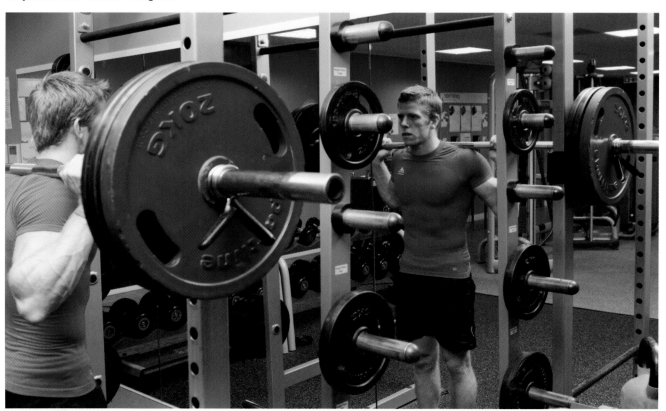

# Why developing maximum strength can improve your running

Tudor Bompa is one of the world's foremost conditioning coaches – he is one of the very few coaches to have trained world/Olympic champions in both power and endurance sports, respectively, the javelin and rowing. As well as being known as the "father of periodisation" (training planning), Bompa has refined over many years his approach to sports conditioning and it is one that rests heavily on the maximum strength (MxS) method – whatever the sport.

The thought of lifting very heavy weights is often not a training priority for the majority of recreational middle and long distance runners. However, if you are a serious runner, perhaps with elite aspirations, then maximum strength weight training could be worth trying. Bompa, when writing about sports performance in general notes that "Higher velocity is

possible only as a result of superior force generation against resistance (i.e. gravity, snow, terrain, profile and water)." He believes that lifting very heavy weights is crucial in order to achieve this higher velocity. Bompa goes on: "A long distance event requires much more than the improvement of force per stride using elements of maximum strength. Athletes must then convert this gain into maximum endurance of long duration so that the force is applied for the entire duration of the race..." (*Strength Training for Sport*: 41). Table 7.2 on pages 80–1, chapter 7, provides an example of such a training programme that focuses around MxS development. Plyometric exercises are great at transferring power and would also be an integral part of this training approach (see page 118).

positioned microcyles involving maximum strength workouts. You could also schedule in strength-endurance and power workouts throughout the training cycle to maintain optimum strength, power and endurance.

If you decide to pursue the development of maximum strength to benefit your running, then it will be best to experiment with both approaches (and others created

by a suitably qualified specialist and/or yourself), i.e. maximum strength development emphasised at the beginning of the training year and a more progressive and consistent approach as shown in the double periodisation model (see page 80).

Also as a recreational runner after a few years of following the types of workouts outlined in this chapter (workouts 1–4), the time could be right to move onto heavier lifting. In order to keep improving you need to constantly stimulate your mind and muscles and the maximum strength method could do just that for you.

## Typical maximum strength workout protocols

- Protocol 1: 4 x 3 x 90% 1RM
- Protocol 2: 3 x 6 x 85% 1RM
- Protocol 3: 8 x 70% 1RM; 2 x 4 x 85% 1RM; 2 x 1 x 95% 1RM 1
- Protocol 4: 4 x 1-2 x 95% 1RM

## How getting stronger makes for faster running

An oft-quoted example is that if a runner is able to increase the force he generates on each stride, he will "shorten" the marathon distance. An average marathon requires 50,000 steps, so if you can increase each and every stride by 1cm, then you would "save" 500m compared to your pre-increased stride length.

To lift such weights dynamically requires considerable physical and mental energy. You'll only have limited amounts of this in reserve to do this, so it's imperative that you are rested and mentally ready ("in the zone") to perform these workouts. Recoveries must be full between sets and reps in order to reduce the effects of fatigue and give you every opportunity of working at 100 per cent intensity. Other lighter weight/body weight exercises could also be included in these workouts after the heavier exercises have been completed.

Note: Ensure you get expert advice on lifting technique and have a spotter/training partner on hand if you are going to attempt these workouts, and only do so after you have developed sufficient preliminary strength over a systematic and progressive training plan.

## Be responsive when planning

As a coach or runner you should be prepared to change your training plans. Runners will adapt at different rates to training. You may also face illness and injury and sources of stress beyond the training environment, which will affect your performance. It will be up to you or your coach to make the adjustments necessary to all aspects of the training programme to achieve peak fitness when it matters. This could mean adding in sessions, varying loadings, scheduling in more rest periods and – in the case of injury/illness – starting further back down the training time-line and progressing a return to full fitness carefully. Experience will help you to decide what to do on many occasions and, therefore, it is important that you keep a record of your training. Your training diary should include information on all your workouts (and races if necessary). Do include subjective comment as well as to how you are feeling and responding to training and competition. Weights lifted, reps completed, as well as mileages, speeds and other measures of performance all need to be included in a way that you can easily track and reference the information.

## Exercise selection for maximum strength

It's best to select exercises that are relevant to running as the mainstays of your running conditioning (whether for maximum or other strength development). These will have a greater positive transference into actual running performance. This is because they mirror/reference movement patterns and balance requirements. This is particularly important with exercise selection when training for maximum strength, as you do no want to waste time and effort on exercises that are unlikely to have a significant effect on improving your running. Suitable exercises would therefore include:

**Lower body**
- Leg presses, single (and double)
- Squats, single and double leg
- Lunges
- Calf raises
- Seated rows
- Bulgarian split squat

## Safer exercises

All exercises are safe providing they are performed with good technique and by the relevantly conditioned. However, when a very heavy weight is added to the equation the potential for injury can be increased. Many conditioning experts would prescribe, for example, the clean and the snatch exercises as key exercises in conditioning greater strength and power. However, their technically demanding nature coupled with the intensity of the loads lifted could increase injury risk. Also the pull on the bar, particularly when it passes hip-height, produces a movement that is quite removed from the dynamics of running. I therefore don't recommend the performance of these and similar exercises, particularly by endurance athletes, and definitely not with very heavy loads.

- Step-ups
- Leg curls
- Split squats

**Upper body**
- Rows, single and double arm

Other, upper body exercises could be included in your training, although for middle and long distance runners these will be less relevant compared to the needs of a sprinter. Rowing exercises, as included in the workouts in this chapter previously, such as the seated row and the prone row, flex and extend the shoulder muscles in a way that is very similar to the running arm action, hence their particular relevance.

## Unilateral exercises

Unilateral exercises, such as single leg squats, single leg presses and lunges and the Bulgarian split squat (see below), are a better option for developing running strength and power compared to those that use both limbs at the same time, for the obvious reason that running is a unilateral activity. Performing, for example, a single leg squat will have a greater potential carry-over to your running than the double leg variant. Having said that, you can perform double leg exercises, for example the leg press, particularly during the initial stages of maximum strength conditioning and with runners who are starting a conditioning programme – doing this will help you to develop the readiness, robustness and strength required for the more intense single leg versions.

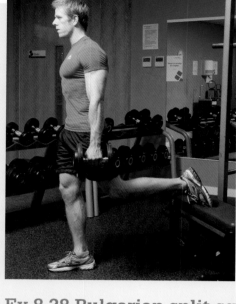

## Ex 8.28 Bulgarian split squat

**Targets**
This exercise targets the glutes, hamstrings and calf muscles and will improve balance.

**How to perform**
Use a squat rack and have a training partner on hand. Stand in front of a sturdy bench. Position the barbell across your shoulders (or hold dumbbells at arm's length). Place the toes of one foot on the bench behind you. Keeping your chest up, while maintaining the natural curves of your spine, bend your front leg to lower your thigh to a position parallel to the ground. Extend your leg to return to the start position. Complete all your reps before swapping legs. Do not let your knee extend past your toes when lifting and lowering to prevent potential damage to the knee joint.

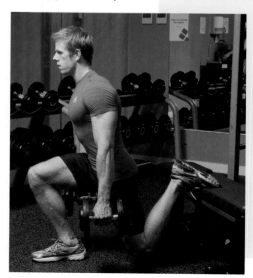

# Plyometric training and running

## Plyometric training – add power to your stride

Whether you run at a sprint or marathon pace you need power and one of the best training ways of developing this most precious commodity is through plyometric (jumping) training. The more dynamic (and as we shall see later, stiffer) your legs become, the more power they are able to supply for each and every stride, whether this be for the 40–45 strides that a male 100m sprinter takes to complete the 100m or the 50,000 required to run a marathon. The increased dynamic ability will increase your stride length and decrease your ground contact times, making you a faster runner.

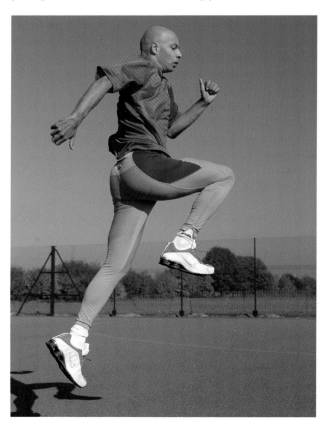

Plyometric exercises are also a great way to channel the strength developed with weights and through the maximum strength method into faster running.

## What is a plyometric exercise? – a reminder

Plyometrics are based on the fact that a concentric (shortening) muscular action is much stronger if it immediately follows an eccentric (lengthening) action of the same muscle. It's a bit like stretching out a coiled spring to its fullest extent and then letting it go. Immense levels of energy will be released in a split second as the spring recoils. Plyometric exercises develop this recoil or, more technically, the "stretch reflex" capacity of muscles. With regular exposure to this training stimulus, muscle fibres will be better able to store and return greater amounts of "elastic" energy.

## Plyometric drills and intensity

### Selecting the best exercises for you

When it comes to selecting the best plyometric exercises for you as a runner, you should consider your running distance and training experience, your level of pre-conditioning (see chapter 1) and your ability to pick up what can be quite complex skills. You also need to factor in previous injuries – those with ankle, knee and back histories need to progress slowly and always be mindful of avoiding further injury (if you are unsure, seek out the services of, for example, a specialist, such as a strength and conditioning coach or a physiotherapist with relevant knowledge). The time in the training year is also important and your workouts should reflect this – intense plyometric workouts should not, for example, take place before important races or track workouts as they could fatigue your leg muscles and/or lead to muscle soreness.

### Plyometric exercise intensity

Single leg exercises are more complex from a skill learning perspective and more stressful than double leg exercises, yet, as we have seen, the former are more relevant to your running needs (as is the case with unilateral weight training exercises). Compare squat jumps to alternate leg bounding ("steps") over 20m, for example – the complexity and speed component of the latter is significantly greater than the former. It's highly unlikely that even a moderately conditioned runner would be able to perform the bounding drill without "collapsing" due to a lack of specific strength. So, always err on the side of caution when selecting plyometric exercises and progress gradually; the best thing to do is to underestimate what you think you can achieve, particularly when you're starting out.

Table 8.2 ranks plyometric exercises by their intensity level (i.e. the stresses they place on the body). It should be noted that in this instance intensity does not mean "less beneficial" – it means the exercises are less

**Table 8.2** Plyometric drills and level of intensity

| Type of plyometric exercise | Exercise no. | Examples | Intensity |
|---|---|---|---|
| Standing based jumps performed on the spot | Ex 8.29 | Split (lunge) jumps | Low |
| | Ex 8.30 | Squat jumps | |
| | Ex 8.31 | Straight leg jumps | |
| | Ex 8.32 | Triangle hops | |
| Low trajectory jumps; pp194–6 | Ex 11.1 (see page 194) | Double footed lateral (side-to-side) line jumps | Low-medium |
| | | Forwards and backwards double-footed jumps over a line (line bounce) | Low-medium |
| | Ex 11.2 (see page 195) | Single leg line hops | Medium |
| | Ex 11.3 (See page 196) | Line bounce | Medium |
| Multiple jumps from standing | Ex 8.33 | 5 x consecutive bounds | Medium |
| | Ex 8.34 | 2 x 6 "bunny" jumps | Medium |
| | Ex 8.35 | Double footed jumps up steps | Medium |
| Eccentric drop and hold drills | Ex 8.36 | Eccentric drop jump | Medium-high |
| | Ex 8.37 | Lateral jump with eccentric landing | |
| Multiple jumps with run-on (use a 5-10m approach to a take-off point) | Ex 8.33 | 3 x 2 hops | High |
| | | 2 x 10 bounds | High |
| Drop/depth jumping (recommended drop height 30–90cm). The higher the height, the greater the strength component; the lower height, the greater the speed. | Ex 8.38 | 2 x 6 jumps – jump down and up | High |
| | Ex 8.38 (variation) | Jump down and hop | Very high |

Note: Medicine ball training is covered in more detail on pages 168–72. Throwing and catching a medicine ball is another form of power training which can develop plyometric strength.

stressful on the body, such as side-to-side jumps, are very effective at developing running power (and protecting against injury), as are the more intense depth jumps. Your plyometric training needs to take in the whole range of intensities (not withstanding your injury history) and variations – doing this will keep your muscles adapting and you will avoid boredom.

> ### Low-intensity plyometrics
> Exercises such as the low trajectory hops, performed laterally and linearly and following a triangular pattern, for example, are all great exercises for strengthening the ankle, knee and hip joints. They require control and precision of movement to perform.

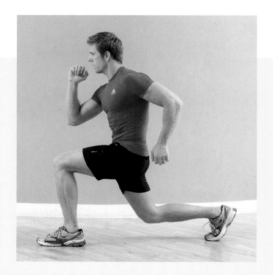

## Ex 8.29 Split jumps

### How to perform
Assume a lunge position. Bend your knees, swing your arms and drive up into the air. Switch your leg position in the air, land and perform another jump. Keep your chest up, core braced and look straight ahead. Land on your forefeet. Complete your designated number of reps and swap legs.

*Do: 3 x 10*

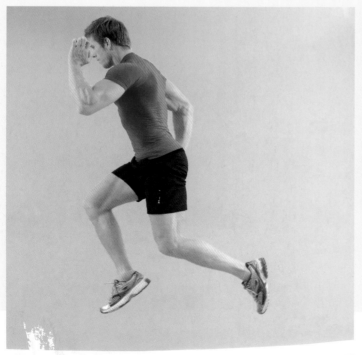

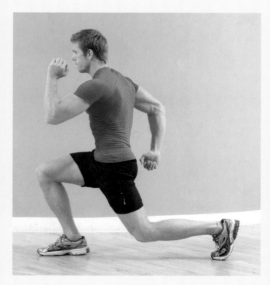

## Ex 8.30 Squat jumps

### How to perform
Bend thighs to a three-quarter squat position and dynamically extend your ankles, knees and hips to jump off the floor. Use your arms to assist your jump power by swinging them backwards and forwards. Land lightly on the balls of the feet and immediately spring into another jump. Brace your core throughout and look straight ahead.

*Do: 3 x 10*

## Ex 8.31 Straight leg jumps

### How to perform
Stand with your feet shoulder-width apart. Slightly flex your knees and jump upwards. Swing your arms in time with your jump. Land with your legs virtually straight and use your calf and ankle muscles to propel yourself into another jump. This is a great exercise for developing ankle power.

*Do: 3 x 10 reps*

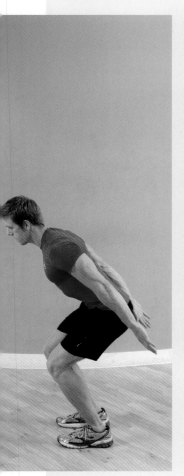
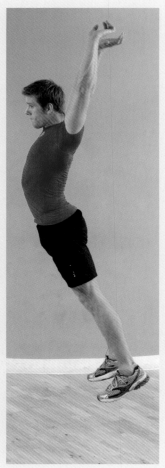
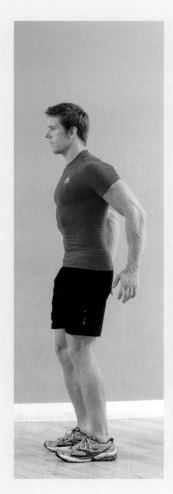
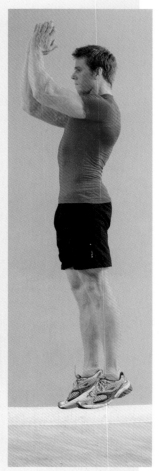

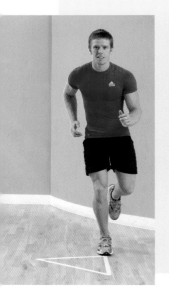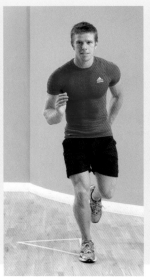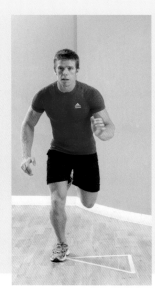

## Ex 8.32 Triangle hops

**How to perform**

Hop to your right using a low trajectory, then immediately forward diagonally and then laterally to approximately where you started from. Continue hopping what is the path of a right-angled triangle for your designated reps and then swap legs and repeat.

*Do: 3 x 8–10 reps*

**Low-medium/medium-intensity plyometrics**

See chapter 11 for more exercises that fall into this category (pages 194–6), and also the exercises described below.

## Ex 8.33 Bounds

**How to perform**

Stand with your feet shoulder-width apart. Leap forward onto one leg and land on your forefoot. Immediately leap forward onto your other leg. Try to stay in the air for as long as you can while keeping your speed. Land light and fast. Swing your non-jumping leg into each bound as dynamically as you can. Keep your chest up and co-ordinate your arms with your legs.

*Do: 4–8 x 20m for medium intensity or high-intensity option: 3 x 2 bounds with run on (see page 118 for a note on plyometric intensity).*

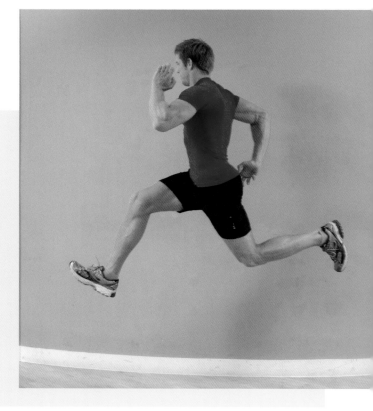

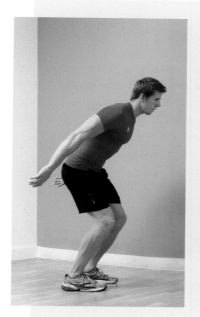
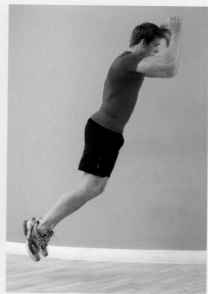
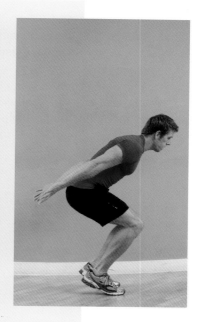

## Ex 8.34 Bunny jumps

### How to perform
Stand with your feet shoulder-width apart. Bend your knees, swing your arms and jump forwards. Land and, without flexing too much at the knees, perform another jump. Land on your feet and keep your head and chest up.

*Do: 3 x 4 reps*

## Ex 8.35 Double footed jumps up steps

### How to perform
Find a suitable run of steps (stadium steps are usually ideal). Bend your knees, swing your arms and leap two steps at a time. Try to move as quickly as possible. Land on your forefeet.

*Do: 2-4 reps*

### Variation
As illustrated: run up the steps taking one or two at a time.

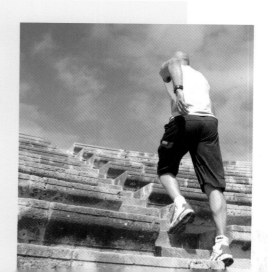

123

### Eccentric drop jumps

Although used in training and subject to research from at least the 1960s onwards, these drills have not been as prevalent in running and other sports training programmes as the other plyometric drills in Table 8.2. This is because eccentric jumping drills focus on the plant and absorption from a jump and are, as such, not truly plyometric (there is no subsequent concentric muscular action, as there would be if the runner was to jump after landing). However, they are advocated as a conditioner of the stretch reflex because they strengthen the absorbency potential of muscles and can develop a more powerful base for the subsequent concentric action. Eccentric training can be of particular use to runners in need of sprint speed.

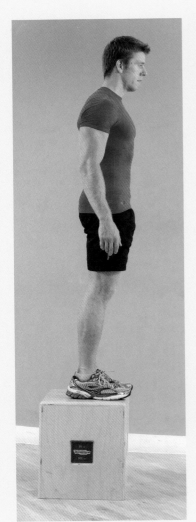

## Ex 8.36 Eccentric drop jump

### How to perform

Stand on top of a sturdy bench (or similar object) 50-70cm high. Step off the bench and land on both feet with only a slight knee bend to 'block' the landing. Land on your forefeet. On impact the muscles of your ankles, knees and hips will be lengthening to absorb the landing (the eccentric muscular action).

*Do: 3 x 4*

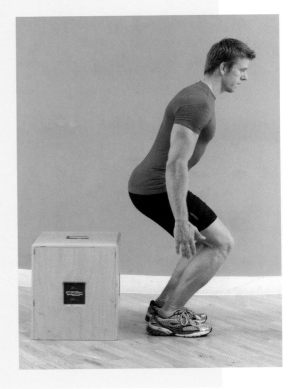

# Ex 8.37 Lateral jump with eccentric landing

## Targets

This exercise, like the majority of the plyometric exercises in this section, targets the thighs, calf and ankle muscles, however, it also focuses on the glute medius (the muscle to the outer portion of your hips). This exercise will be instrumental in developing a running technique that will allow you to exert power in the direction you want, i.e. linearly, without wasteful rotational or lateral movements. These are created by instability that results from weak and non-specifically conditioned core, thigh and hip muscles. The glute medius is crucial in this respect as a stabilising muscle. (Note: Many of the exercises in chapter 9, core training for runners, develop this running-specific strength requirement).

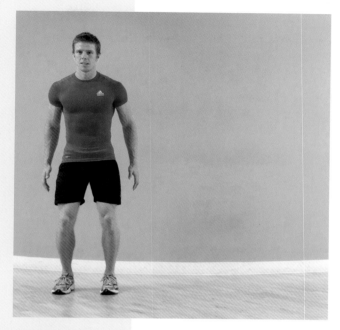

## How to perform

Stand with feet hip-width apart and leap sideways to land on one leg. Slightly flex your leg on landing and brace yourself to root yourself to the spot. If you are unable to do so, persevere as in time you will develop the necessary eccentric strength to be able to do so.

*Do: 3 x 6 on each leg*

## Variations

Similar exercises can be performed by leaping forward onto one leg or two and at various angles and "blocking" the landing. When performing all variations ensure that your foot is in line with your knee/knees of your landing leg/legs – this is particularly important when leaping sideways.

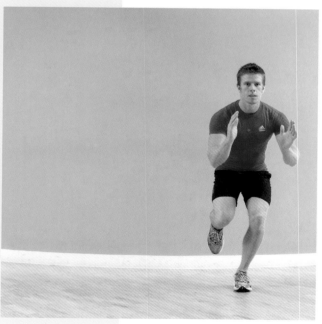

### Depth jumping
Multiple jumps with a run-up

### High–very high intensity plyometrics
As indicated in Table 8.2, these are advanced exercises and require considerable plyometric strength. They should only be performed if you are suitably conditioned. Mark a distance back from your take-off point of 10-15m and then run in at a quick pace to the take-off point to perform the sequence of jumps. You could hop or bound or perform a combination of hops and bounds.

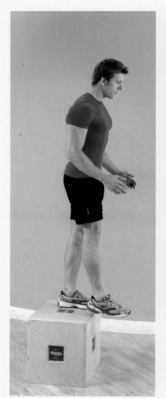
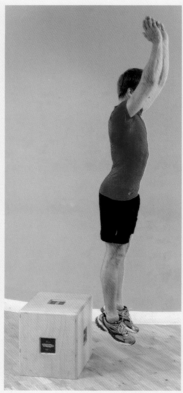
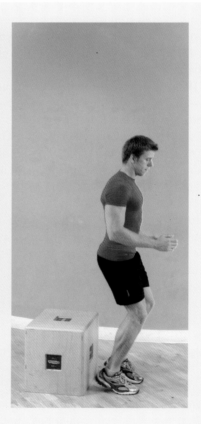

## Ex 8.38 Depth Jumps

### How to perform
Stand on top of a sturdy bench 60–90cm high. Step off to land on two feet and with minimal knee bend jump either upwards or forwards as fast as you can. Use your arms to add to your speed. Keep your chest up and look straight ahead. Land on your forefeet.

### Variations
Multiple jumps can be performed on landing as can single hops and multiple hops, bounds and combinations thereof.

# How to incorporate plyometric training into your run training

Just as you may plan your running training to prepare you for an important race in terms of mileage, intervals, volume and pace, you can follow a similar process with plyometrics. Take a look at the following section to see how this can be achieved.

## Placing plyometrics into a training plan

This "phasing" example is particularly suitable for middle distance track runners, although the principles apply to runners of all speeds and distances.

### Early conditioning phase (autumn/winter)

After a period of basic conditioning and a gradual increase in mileage, you can perform plyometrics to improve muscular endurance. You can achieve this through circuit-style training, including exercises such as split jumps, squat jumps and straight leg jumps (see pages 120–1). You should use normal circuit training

## Muscle soreness and plyometric training

As a runner you need to be aware that plyometric (and eccentric) training is likely to cause muscular soreness even in the well (but not specifically) conditioned. This is also likely if you have never performed these types of exercises and when you include them in your workouts after a lay-off. The soreness is the result of the eccentric muscular action in particular. The resulting "tender to the touch" muscles will soon recover and research indicates that the one session (and it's after-effects) can "inoculate" the body against further potential same-exercise induced soreness for up to a month afterwards.

## Plyometric training tip

Always underestimate what you think you can achieve and don't perform more than 2–3 sets of 4–6 reps in your workouts when starting out – progress very gradually.

protocols, such as high reps, multiple numbers of sets and short recoveries (see pages 130–1 for more details on circuit training). At this stage of general conditioning these exercises will develop low-level power and general running-specific conditioning, as well as specific endurance.

You should progress this plyometric "power endurance" conditioning throughout the endurance building phases. You could perform one to two specific workouts a week and these could also include other body weight exercises, such as press-ups and core exercises (see chapter 9).

### Latter conditioning phases (spring)

Having built up a relevant base of running endurance and plyometric power as the track season approaches (where relevant), there will be a switch to more quality orientated running – more often than not built on anaerobic training methodologies, such as interval training. At this time, your plyometric training can also take on a greater quality aspect. You can increase recoveries between reps and decrease repetitions, so that you are able to perform the exercises more dynamically and with less fatigue impairment.

### Peak season (summer)

When preparing for important races, competitive runners often begin a taper – a period of training designed to bring them to a peak. This will be determined by working back from when they need to be at their best. The key components of their running and running conditioning (weights, plyometrics, etc.) will all aim to intersect during this peak period to produce peak performance – that's speed, speed-endurance, power-endurance and tactical awareness (where relevant). In terms of plyometric training, quality as indicated should become the most important variable and – as in the previous phase – recoveries should be long enough and reps and sets low enough to enable this to be achieved. One or two exercises – in the latter stages of the runner's warm-up or during off-track conditioning workouts – may be all that is needed, as it's a case of maintaining specific condition, rather than developing it.

## Running training tip

Including selected plyometrics in your warm-ups is a great way to gain familiarity with these types of exercises and develop specific running power in a time saving way.

## Plyometric training workout 1

### Time in training year
Preparatory mesocycles

### Purpose
This workout example could form part of the early stages of the preparatory mesocycles – normally the October–December period. It's designed to develop power endurance in a running-specific way. Although this is a circuit and local muscular fatigue will build up as the session progresses, you should always endeavour to move as quickly possible and perform the exercises with the correct technique.

## Plyometric training workout 2

### Time in training year
Preparatory, conversion and competition mesocycles with adjustment to load

### Purpose
This type of workout would be performed in the latter part of the preparatory phase of the macrocycle example – the conversion phase and during the competition-specific macrocycles. The workout could be performed on the same day as a quality track workout, for example, or if time and training circumstance allow, as the second training session of the day.

## Plyometric training workout 1

| Exercise no. | Exercise name | Reps | Sets | Recovery | Training tip |
|---|---|---|---|---|---|
| Ex 8.29 | Split jump | 20 | 4–6 | 30 sec, reducing to 10 sec across the mesocycle (4–6 weeks), with the workout performed 1–3 times a week | Switch leg position as quickly as possible when airborne. Co-ordinate arms with legs. |
| Ex 8.30 | Squat jump | 20 | 4–6 | As above | Make ground contacts as fast and as light as possible. |
| Ex 8.31 | Straight leg jumps | 20 | 4–6 | As above | Keep knee flexion to a minimum, i.e. keep legs virtually straight. |
| Ex 8.55 | Medicine ball wall chest pass | 20 | 4–6 | As above | Move the ball as quickly as possible to and from the wall. |
| Ex 11.2 | Single leg lateral side-to-side jumps | 20 | 4 | As above | Lateral movements are important from an injury avoidance point of view for a runner. |

## Plyometric training workout 2

| Exercise no. | Exercise name | Reps | Sets | Recovery | Comments |
|---|---|---|---|---|---|
| Ex 8.36 | Eccentric depth jumps (box height 30–90cm), two footed landing and jump for height | 6 | 1–4 | 30 sec between jumps and 60 sec between sets | Ground contact speed is the key to these exercises. CNS system fatigue must be monitored, i.e. in terms of slowed reactivity. If this becomes apparent then the session should be truncated or even stopped. |
| (Not illustrated) | Hop from box to hop again (box height 30–90cm) | 4 (alternate legs) | 1–4 | 30 sec between hops and 60 sec between sets | |
| (Not illustrated) | Drop jump to sprint 20m (box height 30–90cm). Step off box to land on two feet then immediately sprint for 20m. | 2 efforts | 1–4 | 60 sec recovery between each rep | Reactivity in terms of performance is again crucial – on landing from the drop jump, the runner must fully engage their neuromuscular system to speed away. |

# Circuit training and running

## Will circuit training make you a better endurance runner?

Circuit training offers a great way to develop both general and specific running strength and local

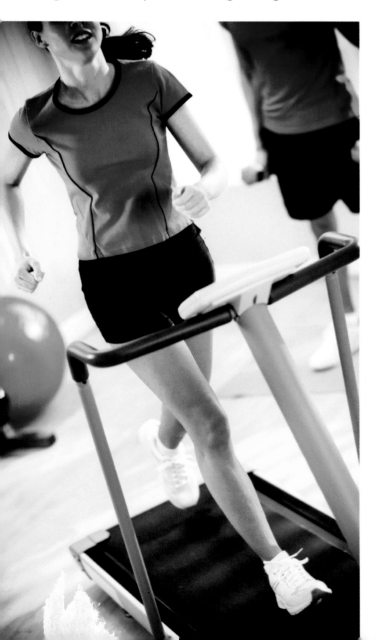

muscular and power endurance. It can also help improve running technique and develop aerobic and anaerobic fitness and protect against injury. In this section, we look at numerous circuit exercises and workout examples.

## Putting a circuit together

There are various ways to construct a circuit, these include:

### Circuit method

This style of circuit requires you to do each different exercise one after the other. For, example, press-ups, followed by squats, followed by the plank and so on. Depending on your level of fitness, the rest periods between exercises and sets can be shorter or longer. The number of circuits, nature and number of exercises will again depend on your level of fitness.

### In-series method

This style of circuit requires you to perform the same exercises in sets before moving onto the next exercise.

For example: 3 x 20 press-ups, followed by 3 x 20 squats, followed by 3 x 30 sec plank, and so on.

In-series circuits are usually tougher than circuit-style ones as the muscle group/groups targeted with each exercise have little recovery before having to work again. Recovery will generally be less than a minute and could be as little as 10 seconds. Therefore, if you are new to circuit training, it's best to progress to this type of circuit over time by progressively increasing the volume of circuit-style circuits first.

### Circuit resistance training (CRT)

This type of circuit specifically uses weights (whether this be through Powerbags, barbells, kettlebells and medicine balls or similar). In reality they are a form of weight training. The workouts described previously in this chapter on pages 96–117 are, in reality, circuit resistance workouts. A distinction between CRT and weight training can be made when lifting weights in excess of 60 per cent of 1RM with reduced reps and longer recoveries. These types of workouts develop power and maximum strength. CRT circuit workouts (in-series and circuit-style) squarely aim at developing strength and power endurance – they use high numbers of reps and sets and short recoveries.

### Aerobic/anaerobic circuit training

These types of circuits include a specific cardio-vascular (CV) element between circuits and/or exercises. Although a circuit is in itself cardiovascular developing in nature, depending on its design a greater aerobic and/or anaerobic pay-off can be added. For example, you could include running, rowing or cycling between exercises or at the end of each circuit. Generally speaking, if these intervals are more than a couple of minutes and are performed at moderate effort levels, for example, around 60–70 per cent of maximum heart rate (MHR), then the circuit will have a greater aerobic, rather than anaerobic, element. However, if you were to perform a 30-second exercise sprint between each circuit exercise then the outcome would definitely be anaerobic.

> Aerobic circuit example: Complete 4 x 20 squats, press-ups and plank (with 20 sec hold) circuit style with 10 sec between exercises and 2 minutes of easy running at the end of each circuit.

### Plyometric circuit training

Emphasising plyometric exercises, such as squat jumps and straight leg jumps, can create very dynamic circuits. These circuits are very intense and should only be performed by the well and specifically conditioned. As circuits develop, local and general muscular fatigue technique will be impaired, hence the need for you to be used to and able to withstand the forces that plyometric circuits generate.

### Peripheral heart action training

PHA circuits require you to perform exercises in a sequence that moves from upper body to lower body and so on. This transition will increase energy expenditure as the body has to divert blood flow constantly.

For example: 20 of each of squats, shoulder press, lunges, upright rows, calf raises, sprint arm action and single leg squats.

You would move straight on from one exercise to the next and may or may not (depending on the level of your fitness) take a rest at the end of each circuit of exercises.

## How to progress a circuit

There are numerous ways to progress a circuit in terms of its intensity, volume and effects. As we have seen, circuit-style circuits are easier, at least when starting a circuit training programme, compared to in-series ones. This is because the former allows the muscle/muscles being worked greater recovery before you work them specifically again (unless, of course, an exercise that works the same muscles is included immediately afterwards, for example, squats followed by lunges).

Aerobic/anaerobic CV circuit training is perhaps the toughest of all the options for runners as it can tax all energy systems – aerobic, anaerobic – and develop lactate tolerance, VO2max and local muscular endurance and power. Lactate is a chemical produced in the body at all times, its levels increase with increased exercise intensity. At a point of intensity the rate of its production will exceed the rate of its clearance and re-use for energy production and energy creating switches from aerobic to anaerobic. It's also at this point that it's molecular structure changes and it turns into lactic acid. Circuit training can increase muscles' lactate usage and tolerance and increase their ability to process this chemical, before it becomes lactic, thus increasing endurance.

Circuit training is also good for developing increased will-power and pain tolerance – vital qualities for successful endurance running.

# Circuits for runners

In the following circuits you'll see that a number of progression options have been provided, which will help you to design and develop your own circuit training workouts in future, so that you can increase your fitness over time. Exercise descriptions are provided for exercises that you may be less familiar with.

You should use the options provided for each of the circuits, together with reps and sets, for **guideline purposes only** to shape your workouts, progressively and in a way that is specific to your level of fitness and time in your training year/period. The second circuit contains plyometric exercises – substitute these with a less intense option as necessary.

# General running condition circuit 1

**Suitable for**

Option 1 (see table) runners of all levels to use throughout the training year (option 2 – see table – is the more advanced option for those new to circuit training, and should be progressed to over time after a high level of strength endurance has been developed by using option 1 to develop appropriate fitness).

**Progression**

Gradually build up the number of sets and reps performed and reduce the recovery time.

**Note:** A range of reps is provided – select according to your level of fitness and time in your training (the same applies to recovery, options and sets).

## General running condition circuit 1

| Exercise no. | Exercise name | Reps | Sets | Recovery |
|---|---|---|---|---|
| Ex 8.39 | Squats | 20–60 | 2–6 | |
| Ex 8.40 | Press-ups | 10–40 Substitute press-ups from knees if you are unable to complete full press-ups | 2–6 | |
| Ex 8.19 (see page 108) | Plank | 10–45 sec hold | 2–6 | **Option 1: Perform exercises circuit style – 30 sec between exercises, 60 sec between circuits** |
| Ex 8.41 | Walking lunges | 20–40 | 2–6 | |
| Ex 8.42 | Hip bridge | 10–30 | 2–6 | **Option 2: In-series – 20 sec between exercises, and straight through sets** |
| Ex 8.43 | Side plank | 10–30 sec hold each side | 2–6 | |
| Ex 8.44 | Marching high knees on spot | 40–80 ground contacts | 2–6 | |
| Ex 8.45 | Seated sprint arm action | 20–60 sec (depending on your fitness) | 2–6 | |

# Exercise descriptions

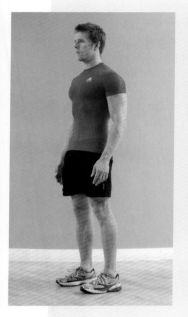
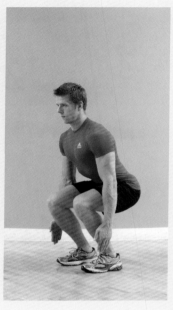

## Ex 8.39 Squat

**Targets**
This exercise targets the glutes and thighs.

**How to perform**
Stand with feet just beyond shoulder-width apart. Bend knees to lower thighs to close to a 90-degree angle to the ground. Ensure that you keep your knees behind your toes and prevent any lateral or rotational movements. Push back through your heels and extend your hips near to the top of the movement to return to the start position. You can hold your arms by your sides, place your hands on your hips, or hold them straight out and parallel to the ground. The latter option will, for many people, make squatting easier as it helps maintain the natural curves of the spine – which is a requirement of the exercise.

## Ex 8.40 Press-up

**Targets**
This exercise targets the chest, shoulders, triceps and core.

**How to perform**
Assume a prone position, legs extended and hands below shoulders. Extend your arms to lift your body from the floor, maintaining a straight line from the back of your shoulders, across your bottom and to your heels. Lower your chest to within a few centimetres of the floor. Extend your arms to complete one rep. Substitute press-ups from the knees if you are unable to complete full press-ups.

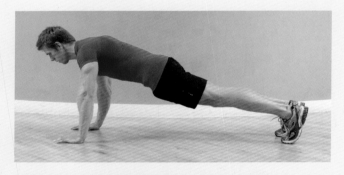
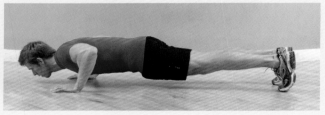

## Ex 8.41 Walking lunge

### Targets
This exercise targets the thighs and calf muscles.

### How to perform
Take a large step forward into a lunge, allowing your front thigh to reach a position near parallel to the ground. Immediately step through into another lunge, making sure not to elevate too much when transitioning from one lunge to the next – try to "push through your hips". Co-ordinate your arms with your legs – that's opposite arm to leg – and keep your chest elevated throughout. If you do not have a lot of space to complete this exercise, lunge forwards and backwards on the spot alternating lead leg.

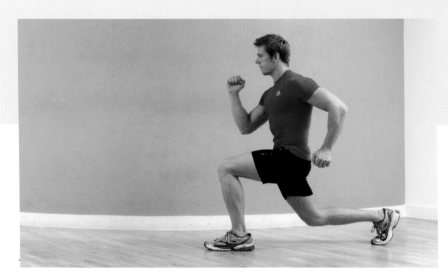

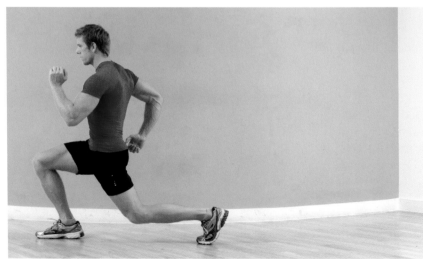

## Ex 8.42 Hip bridge

### Targets
This exercise targets the hamstrings and bottom.

### How to perform
Lie on your back with your hands by your side and feet just beyond hip-width apart. Press your heels into the ground and lift your hips. Hold this extended position for a two count before lowering and repeating.

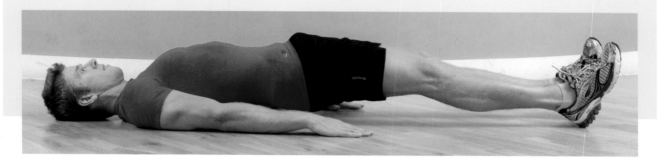

## Ex 8.43 Side plank

### Targets
This exercise targets the core (in particular the sides).

### How to perform
Lie on your side with your elbow under your shoulder and forearm facing forward. Keeping your body in alignment, stack your hips on top of each other and rest your other arm along the top of your body. Push up to lift your body off the ground and hold.

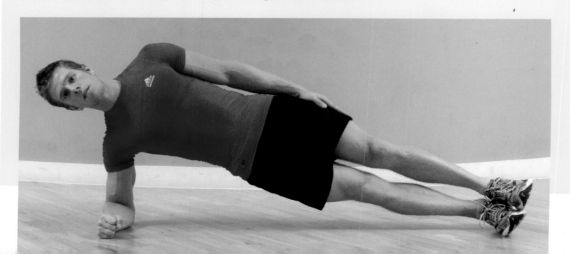

## Ex 8.44 Marching high knees

**Targets**

This exercise targets the hip flexors (muscles at the top of thighs), calf muscles, quadriceps and core.

**How to perform**

Stand tall and lift and lower each leg (bending at the knee) to a thigh-parallel-to-the-ground position. Co-ordinate your arms with your legs and keep your chest elevated. Focus on picking each leg up and driving it back to the ground. Contact the ground on your forefeet.

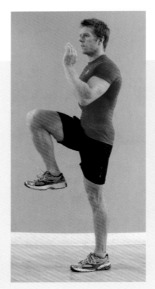
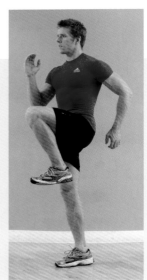

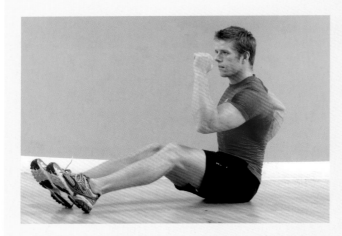

## Ex 8.45 Seated sprint arm action

**Targets**

This exercise targets the shoulders, upper back and core.

**How to perform**

Assume a seated position with your legs extended and torso upright. Begin to pump your arms backwards and forwards as if running. Your front arm's hand should reach a position near to your eye level, with the rear upper arm nearing or reaching a position parallel to the ground behind you.

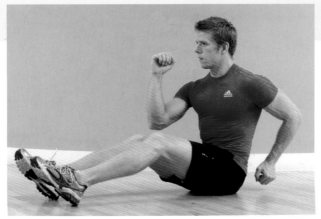

# General running conditioning circuit 2

**Suitable for**

As general running conditioning circuit 1 (see page 132), but the inclusion of plyometric exercises makes it more dynamic. Ensure that you are specifically conditioned to perform this circuit.

Note: A range of reps is provided – select according to your level of fitness and time in your training (the same applies to recovery, options and sets).

| General running conditioning circuit 2 | | | | |
| --- | --- | --- | --- | --- |
| Exercise no. | Exercise name | Reps | Sets | Recovery |
| Ex 8.30 (see page 121) | Squat jump | 10–30 | 2–6 | |
| Ex 8.46 | Triceps dip | 20–40 | 2–6 | |
| Ex 4.9 (see page 43) | Plank with leg raise | 1–4 with 10–30 sec holds for each leg | 2–6 | |
| Ex 8.29 (see page 120) | Split jump | 10–20 (L and R) | 2–6 | **Option 1: Perform exercises circuit style, 20 sec between exercises, 60 sec between circuits** |
| Ex 8.47 | One leg dynamic bridge | 10–30 (L and R) | 2–6 | |
| Ex 8.4 (see page 97) | Calf raises (performed without added resistance) | 20–60 | 2–6 | **Option 2: In-series style, 15 sec between exercises and straight through sets** |
| Ex 8.48 (see page 139) | Plank with torso twist | 10–30 (alternate legs) | 2–6 | |
| Ex 8.31 (see page 121) | Straight leg jump | 10–20 | 2–6 | |

## Exercise descriptions

### Ex 8.46 Triceps dip

**Targets**
This exercise targets the triceps.

**How to perform**
Using a sturdy bench or chair, face away from it and place the palms of your hands on it, with fingers facing forwards and legs extended. Bend your arms to lower your bottom towards the floor then push dynamically back up to the start position. For a less advanced option bend your knees.

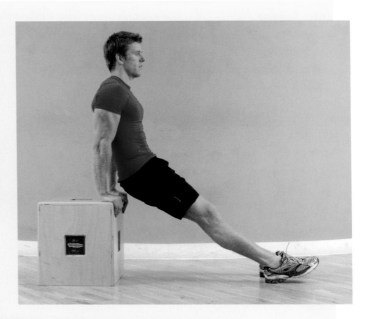

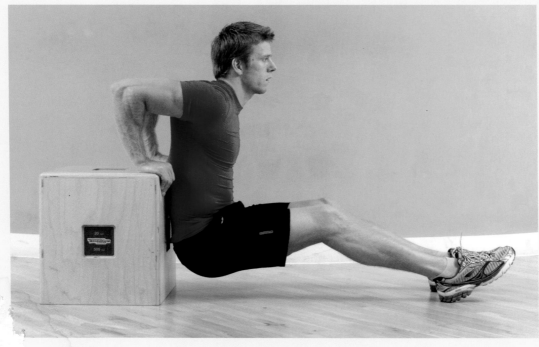

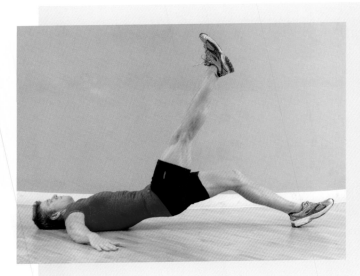

## Ex 8.47 One leg dynamic bridge

### Targets
This exercise targets the core, bottom and hamstrings.

### How to perform
Lie on the floor and position your upper arms so that they are parallel to your shoulders with your forearms at right angles and hands flat on the floor. Keeping your pelvis square, press your heels into the ground to lift your hips off the floor. Set yourself and then lift one leg up as far as your flexibility allows. Lower under control and repeat. Complete all reps on one side before swapping legs.

## Ex 8.48 Plank with torso twist

### Targets
This exercise targets the shoulders, hip flexors and core.

### How to perform
Assume a press-up start position, i.e. with arms extended. Lift one leg off the floor and rotate your body as you take the knee of the elevated leg under your body toward its opposite elbow. Bend your arms slightly as you do this. Extend your arms and return the leg to the start position and then repeat to the other side.

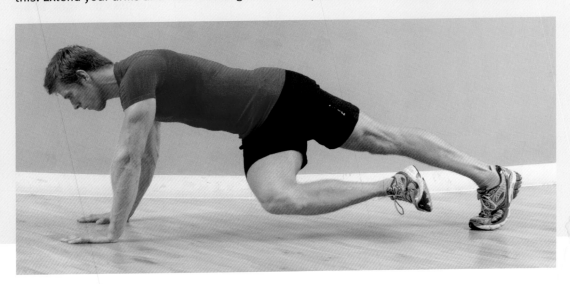

# Circuit resistance training circuits for runners (CRT)

Circuit resistance training (CRT) offers great potential for the runner. As we have seen, it typically combines relatively light weight training exercises (50–60 per cent of 1RM) and body weight exercises. Because of the weights elements it can be more effective at increasing lean muscle mass and creating a greater calorific and CV effect compared to more standard body weight exercises (see also power endurance weight training page 105).

## CRT circuit 1
**Suitable for**
All levels and speeds of runners

Note: A range of reps is provided – select according to your level of fitness and time in your training (the same applies to recovery, options and sets).

### CRT circuit 1

| Exercise no. | Exercise name | Reps | Sets | Recovery |
|---|---|---|---|---|
| Ex 8.10 (see page 102) | Squat with barbell, Powerbag or holding dumbbells at arm's length | 10–30 | 2–6 | |
| Ex 8.13 (see page 104) | Sprint arm action with light dumbbells | 20–40 | 2–6 | |
| Ex 8.19 (see page 108) | Plank | 1–4 reps with 10–30 sec hold | 2–6 | **Option 1: Perform exercises circuit style, 30 sec between exercises, 60 sec between circuits** |
| Ex 8.49 | Lunge with barbell/Powerbag or holding dumbbells at arm's length | 10–20 (L and R) | 2–6 | |
| Ex 8.5 (see page 98) | Swiss ball hamstring curl | 10–30 | 2–6 | **Option 2: Perform exercises in-series, 20 sec between exercises and sets and 60 sec between sets of the exercises** |
| Ex 8.4 (see page 97) | Calf raises with barbell/Powerbag or holding dumbbells at arm's length | 20–60 | 2–6 | |
| Ex 8.50 | Goblet Squat | 20 alternate legs (dependent of fitness) | 2–6 | |
| Ex 8.51 | Single leg squat with barbell/Powerbag or holding dumbbells at arm's length | 10–30 (dependent of fitness) | 2–6 | |

# Exercise descriptions

### Ex 8.49 Lunge holding dumbbells at arm's length or with barbell/Powerbag

**Targets**
This exercise targets the glutes, thighs and calf muscles.

**How to perform**
Hold the dumbells at arm's length. Stand with feet shoulder-width apart. Take a large step forward into a lunge and bend both knees to 90 degrees. Push back through the heel of your front leg to return to the start position. Keep your chest elevated and your core braced throughout. Lunge forwards with your opposite leg and continue exercise.

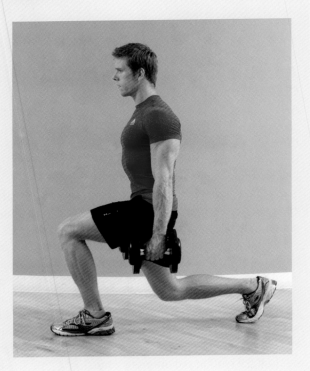

### Ex 8.50 Goblet Squat

**Targets**
This exercise targets the glutes, thighs, arms and core (the latter as you brace to support the weight).

**How to perform**
Take hold of a dumbbell or kettlebell in two hands and support it across your chest. Stand with your feet shoulder-width apart. Keeping your chest up, bend your knees to a 90-degree angle and then push back up through your heels to return to the starting position.

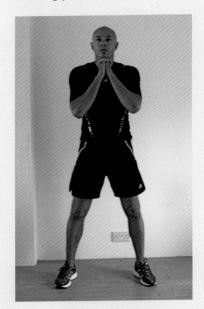

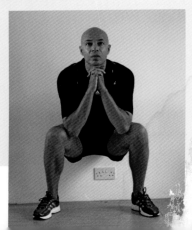

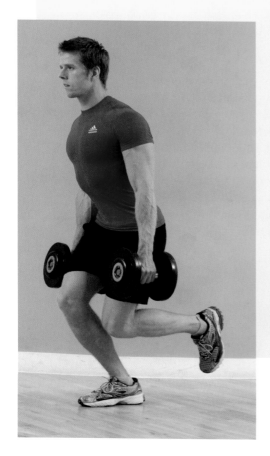

## Ex 8.51 Single leg squat (dumbbell version)

### Targets
This exercise targets the thighs and glutes and promotes balance.

### How to perform
Hold dumbbells at arm's length. Stand with feet shoulder-width apart and bend one leg so that its heel is close to your bottom. Bend your standing knee and lower to as near to 90 degrees as possible, keeping your heel in contact with the ground and maintaining the natural curves of your spine throughout. Push back up through your heel to return to the start position, extending your hips at the top of the movement. Focus on dropping your bottom to the floor over your heel. Complete reps and swap legs.

### Progression
Extend your non squatting leg straight out in front of you. This exercise is known as a "pistol squat" and also strengthens the hip flexors of the extended leg as they work to hold the leg in place.

## Aerobic/anaerobic training circuits for runners

As we have seen, aerobic circuits include a specific cardiovascular (CV) activity or activities – depending on the pace they are performed at and your fitness level, the overall effect of the circuit will be either more (or less) aerobic or anaerobic targeted.

The CV aspect can be included at the end of each circuit or between selected or every exercise (numerous circuit examples are provided in this section).

The duration and intensity of the CV parts can be varied in a multitude of ways, for example, 30 seconds all-out effort shuttle sprints or exercise bike sprints or more sedate 3-minute efforts, or even 400m or 800m reps if performing the workout on a running track (or marked area). You could also use heart rate to control the CV element (and the overall level of the circuit, if so desired, i.e working to different zones).

### Get creative – design your own workouts
In this and other sections of this chapter and book I have described numerous exercises that you can use to construct your own circuit and weights workouts. You should select exercises that are relevant to you and your level of fitness, what equipment you have available and the time in the training year.

# Circuits can boost VO$_2$max

VO$_2$max is a measure of the body's maximum oxygen processing capacity and can be increased by aerobic/anaerobic circuit training. In fact, according to research, it increased by as much as 18 per cent in the participants in a circuit that involved 3 minutes of aerobic activity followed by five weights exercises (using weights of 40–50 per cent of 1RM) performed five times. This totalled 45 minutes of continuous effort).

## Aerobic/anaerobic circuit 1: Variable speed interval circuit

**Suitable for**
Runners with an advanced level of relevant fitness

Note: This is an advanced circuit option because of the running speeds required between exercises. However, it can be made easier by adjusting the duration and intensity of the running efforts. For example, all runs could be performed at a comfortable aerobic pace – 60 per cent of maximum heart rate or 50 per cent speed level.

### Aerobic/anaerobic circuit 1: Variable speed interval circuit

| Exercise no. | Exercise name | Reps/time on | Sets | Recovery |
|---|---|---|---|---|
| Ex 8.41 (see page 134) | Walking lunge | 30 sec | 2–6, depending on level of fitness | The run elements (time and speed) determine the outcome of the circuit, i.e. the faster the runs, the more anaerobic the circuit; the slower the runs, the more aerobic the circuit |
| | Run at 60% speed | 60 sec | | |
| Ex 8.19 (see page 108) | Plank | 30-sec hold | | |
| | Run at 70% speed | 60 sec | | |
| Ex 8.39 (see page 133) | Squats | 30 sec | | |
| | Run at 70% speed | 90 sec | | |
| Ex 8.45 (see page 136) | Sprint arm action | 40 reps | | |
| | Run at 80% speed | 90 sec | | |
| Ex 8.4 (see page 97) | Calf raises | 40 reps | | |
| | Run at 70% speed | 90 sec | | |
| Ex 8.52 | Treadmills | 30 sec | | |
| | Run at 70% speed | 60 sec | | |
| Ex 8.31 (see page 121) | Straight leg jumps | 30 sec | | |
| | Run at 60% speed | 60 sec | | |

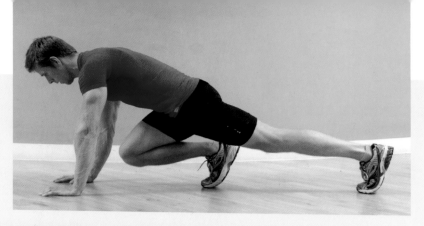

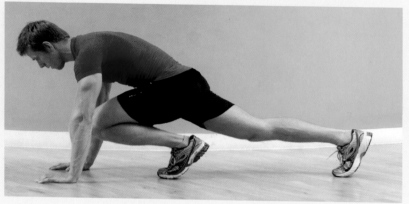

## Ex 8.52 Treadmills

### Targets
This exercise targets the shoulders, core and hip flexors.

### How to perform
Assume a press-up start position. Maintaining the natural curves of your spine and keeping this and your bottom near parallel to the ground, alternate pulling each leg in toward your chest and back to the start positions. Your legs should pump backwards and forwards while your upper body remains relatively stable.

## Aerobic/anaerobic circuit 2: Out and back anaerobic circuit

### Suitable for
Runners with an intermediate/advanced level of relevant fitness. Although this circuit can be done individually, it's a great one to do with other runners – getting competitive will really up the intensity and increase your strength and fitness levels.

### Purpose
To develop high-end anaerobic fitness and lactate tolerance (will also improve VO2max).

### How to perform
Use cones (or other suitable objects) to mark out a distance of 20m. The exercises will be performed at one end (the start), after the completion of each run of 20m backwards and forwards (total distance 40m).

The out and back circuit is best performed on a number of sets-completed basis. Two runners could compete against each other to finish the circuit first, or two or more pairs of runners could perform the workout as a relay. If the first option is performed (i.e. 1 vs 1), then the only "recovery" will be the 20m out and back part. If performed in pairs, then the time it takes for each "partner" to perform their exercises and run backwards and forwards will be the recovery.

Due to the potential speed and competitive nature of the workout there will be a tendency to perform the exercises without the best technique, as they are "rushed" to either catch the other person/team or maintain a lead. Therefore a) it's best to select exercises that have little room for too much "cheating" and b) have a coach on hand to try to ensure technique remains within reasonable parameters. Exercises must, of course, be performed safely.

**Exercises suitable for inclusion in the Out and Back circuit:**

- Ex 8.40 Press-up – target, chest to floor (see page 133)
- Ex 8.39 Squat – target, thighs parallel to floor (see page 133)
- Ex 8.29 Split (lunge) jumps (see page 120)
- Ex 8.52 Treadmills (see page 144)
- Ex 8.52 Treadmills, but bringing knees to the outside of same side elbow
- Ex 8.46 Triceps dip (see page 138)

## Fartlek and circuit training for runners

Many runners will use fartlek-style training in their workouts. Fartlek is Swedish for "speed play". Essentially, when you are out on a run, you decide what pace to run at and for how long. You may decide, for example, to run between two trees 300m apart at a fast pace and then jog easily for 2 minutes, then sprint up a steep incline for 40m and so on.

Numerous circuit training exercises can be incorporated within a fartlek. You could use park benches to perform step-ups or triceps dips or feet elevated press-ups, for example.

## Using circuits to build speed

With its emphasis on developing strength-endurance, it's not often readily appreciated that circuit training can be used to develop high-end speed and speed-endurance and power. Speed-endurance is required by middle distance track runners, for example, who need to maintain fast paces for moderate periods of time. This effort places reliance on the anaerobic energy system. Although speed circuits are particularly suited to the sprinter, they can also benefit endurance runners, as they will lay a foundation of running-specific strength and power.

When you perform a circuit designed to develop speed, the key relevant training variable is quality, i.e.

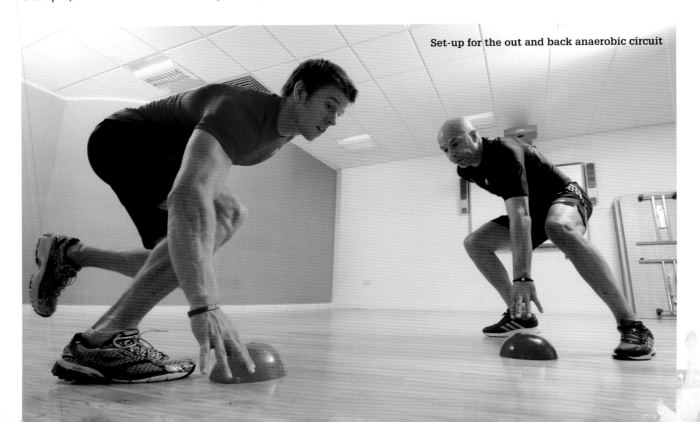

Set-up for the out and back anaerobic circuit

the exercises must be performed quickly and with limited fatigue. Therefore, you'll need to take long enough recoveries. Additionally, you should control the number of reps/time on each exercise to allow you to continue the dynamic movement with only limited disruption created by fatigue.

| Speed-developing running circuit | | |
| --- | --- | --- |
| **Exercise no.** | **Exercise name** | **Reps/time** |
| Ex 8.13 (See page 104) | Sprint arm action – from lunge position | See below P110 for a specific circuit time, rep and format progression over a mesocycle for this workout |
| Ex 3.6 (see page 31) | Single leg cycling | |
| Ex 8.11 (see page 102) | Alternate knee to elbow crunch ("chinnies") | |
| Ex 8.53 | Single leg speed hops on spot | |
| Ex 8.54 | Seated sprint arm action | |
| Ex 3.9 (see page 34) | Wall leg drives | |
| Ex 8.19 (see page 108) | Plank | |
| Ex 8.55 | Medicine ball wall chest pass | |

# Exercises descriptions

## Ex 8.53 Single leg speed hops on the spot

**Targets**
This exercise targets the leg and ankle muscles.

**Purpose**
Fast running requires very fast foot contacts and reactivity. Performing this exercise will help condition this reaction.

**How to perform**
From standing hop into the air from one foot, land and react as quickly as you can to perform another hop. Focus on making your ground contacts light, fast and as reactive as possible. Don't hop too high. Co-ordinate your arms with your legs – that's moving opposite arm to leg – and keep your chest elevated.

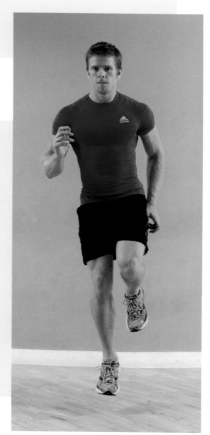

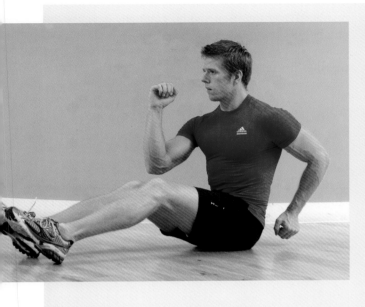

# Ex 8.54 Seated sprint arm action

**Targets**
This exercise targets the core and shoulders.

**Purpose**
The main difference between this and the variant performed from the lunge position are the forces that the core is subject to. The seated position provides a less stable base, through which greater forces will pass through the trunk, resulting in twisting movements. This means that you'll need increased core strength to withstand these forces.

**How to perform**
Sit on the floor with legs extended. Keep your trunk upright and look straight ahead. Pump your arms backwards and forwards as if sprinting, maintaining an approximate 90-degree angle at the elbows.

# Ex 8.55 Medicine ball wall chest pass

**Targets**
This exercise targets the chest, shoulders and core.

**Purpose**
Arm speed and power are crucial for sprinting – this exercise will develop plyometric power in the shoulders and chest.

**How to perform**
Stand close to a wall holding a light (2–5kg) medicine ball. "Move" the ball as fast as possible as you chest pass it against the wall. Brace your core and don't stand too far away from the wall.

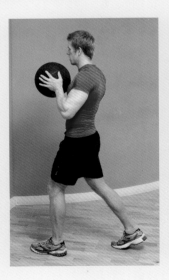
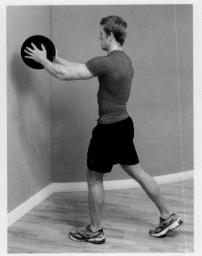

# How to progress a circuit – example

Using a speed circuit, let's see how we can progress circuit training. This depends on the manipulation of the training variables – rest, quantity and quality (see pages 69–71). Keep in mind that the intensity and effect of the session will also depend to a large degree on your prior level of conditioning and your specific fitness and willpower. Greater or fewer quality reps may, therefore, be possible.

All circuits should start with a manageable amount of reps and sets (even if you initially underestimate this number). Over time you should gradually increase the number of reps or the time spent on each station. An example of an eight-week progression is provided for the specific running speed circuit. You should perform two workouts a week.

## Recovery between exercises

You should initially perform the circuit in circuit style (see page 130) and you should leave a long enough recovery to allow you to perform the exercises as fast as possible without significant impairment caused by fatigue. Advanced exercisers could perform the circuit

| Example speed circuit progression | | | | | | | | | |
|---|---|---|---|---|---|---|---|---|---|
| Exercise no. | Exercise/week | 1 | 2 | 3 | 4 | 5 | 6 | 7 | 8 |
| Ex 8.13 (See page 104) | Sprint arm action with dumbbells | 2 x 10 sec | 2 x 12 sec | 2 x 15 sec | 3 x 12 sec | 3 x 14 sec | 3 x 16 sec | 3 x 18 sec | 4 x 15 sec |
| Ex 3.6 (see page 31) | Leg cycling | 2 x 15 left and right | 2 x 18 | 2 x 20 | 3 x 16 | 3 x 18 | 3 x 20 | 3 x 20 | 4 x 16 |
| Ex 8.11 (see page 102) | Alternate knee to elbow crunch ("chinnies") | 2 x 15 | 2 x 18 | 2 x 20 | 3 x 16 | 3 x 18 | 3 x 20 | 3 x 20 | 4 x 16 |
| Ex 8.53 (see page 146) | Hops | 2 x 10 Left and right | 2 x12 | 2 x 15 | 3 x 12 | 3 x 14 | 3 x 16 | 3 x 16 | 4 x 14 |
| Ex 8.54 (see page 147) | Seated sprint arms | 2 x 10 sec | 2 x 15 sec | 2 x 20 sec | 3 x 20 sec | 3 x 20 sec | 3 x 25 sec | 3 x 30 sec | 4 x 25 sec |
| Ex 3.9 (see page 34) | Wall leg drives | 2 x 10 | 2 x 12 | 2 x 15 | 3 x 12 | 3 x 14 | 3 x 16 | 3 x 18 | 4 x 15 |
| Ex 8.19 (See page 108) | Plank | 2 x 20 sec | 2 x 25 sec | 2 x 28 sec | 3 x 20 sec | 3 x 25 sec | 3 x 25 sec | 3 x 25 sec | 4 x 25 sec |
| Ex 8.55 | Medicine ball chest pass | 2 x 20 | 2 x 25 | 2 x 30 | 3 x 25 | 3 x 30 | 3 x 30 | 3 x 30 | 4 x 25 |

in-series, taking 20–30 seconds' recovery between sets of exercises and the transition to each exercise, i.e. from the sprint arm lunge to leg drives and so on.

You should consider the progressions for the circuit given – they have been designed to gradually enhance condition while in this case developing speed and speed-endurance over time. You'll note that some exercises are not progressed as much as others in terms of reps. This is because some are tougher and will result in greater fatigue. You should account for this when progressing your circuits. Not only should you account for the fact that each exercise in this and any other circuit will have its own specific level of fatigue creation, but you will also be better naturally and historically at certain exercises. You may, for example, find press-ups easier than triceps dips. You should therefore also factor this into the construction and progression of your circuit workouts. Returning to the speed circuit, by week 8, you should have sufficient speed-endurance to complete all exercises with lightening speed.

## Further applications of the speed circuit

It would make sense for a middle distance runner to include this circuit into their training prior to the track season. If you are a more "everyday" runner, you could use the workout at the start of the training year to improve power, technique and reactivity.

# Other forms of resistance running training

## Hill training

Hill training will strengthen your running muscles very specifically, as well as having equally positive benefits for your aerobic and anaerobic fitness, depending on how you structure the session. Shorter hill reps are a very useful "channelling" training method in that they can assist the transference of strength developed in the weights rooms, perhaps through the maximum strength method (see page 115) more directly into your running.

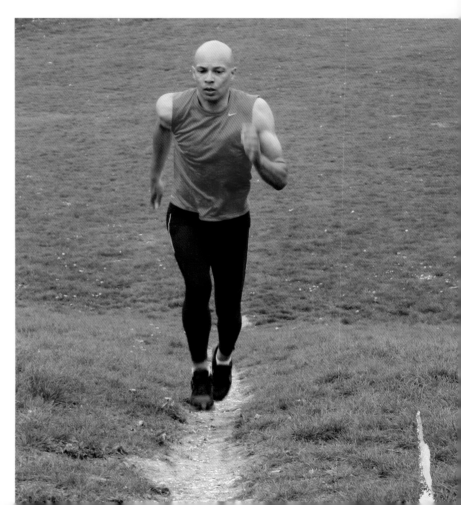

In terms of developing running-specific speed, strength and power, the distance and grade of the hill should be kept relatively short and slight – 50–100m and less than 6 per cent respectively (you could use steeper and longer gradients to develop greater aerobic/anaerobic condition, for example, and as a means to develop specific terrain "experience" if you are planning a race with similar conditions). If you want your hill work to have the utmost chance of improving your specific running speed, you should keep your recoveries relatively long – it's best that fatigue does not affect your ability to run fast and fluently. You should therefore use recoveries of 2–4 minutes for

distances up to 100m to allow for quality running, with the total number of runs being in the 6–10 range.

When running faster than 80 per cent of maximum speed in particular, you will increase the contractile capabilities of your muscles and their fast twitch motor units. You'll have to put in the mental effort to do this and over time and with repeated use you'll turn the key to unlocking greater fast twitch muscle horsepower – or more simply put, your speed!

## Hill running technique

A powerful arm and leg drive are crucial for speedy hill reps. Follow these technique tips:

- Legs should assume a piston-like action, especially when initially accelerating up the hill to generate speed.
- The "work" should be done behind the body to "drive" you up the hill.
- Maintain a forward lean of the trunk for the first 20m or so to assist the drive.
- Drive your arms powerfully backwards and forwards to assist acceleration.
- Make your foot strikes on your forefeet.
- Once into your running keep your chest elevated and look ahead of you (not at the ground).

## Downhill running

Just as you can run uphill, you can run downhill. Downhill running is, however, a much less used component of runners' training, particularly for middle and long distance runners – sprinters will be more likely to use such methods.

Sprinting down grades of 1–2 degrees is known as over-speed training (other over-speed methods include bungee harness running). However, research is inconclusive as to whether these methods do specifically enhance running speed. The grade has to be slight, as too steep a grade will a) negatively affect running dynamics and b) result in a situation where the runner does not "fire" their muscles to move quicker – rather they will let the momentum of the downhill take

### Steeper hills – ascents and descents

On occasion, you can use steeper hill ascents – the benefits of these will be more neural in terms of fast twitch motor unit recruitment and strength orientated, rather than technical. This is because normal running biomechanics can be negatively affected by the gradient. You will need to utilise a lot of mental energy to move yourself powerfully up the hill. It's a bit like what's required of maximum strength weight training – a focused supply of neural energy will be required to develop the power needed to lift the heavy weight and, in this case, overcome the resistance of the steep hill climb.

Longer (and steeper) hill reps (100m+) with shorter, for example, jog-back recoveries can be used for the development of greater heart and lung capacity during appropriate times in the training cycle. These could generate high levels of lactate and lactic acid and boost lactate threshold and tolerance, if the runs were performed fast and the recoveries were kept purposely short.

them to higher speeds, rather than put in the mental effort to do it themselves.

If you try over-speed downhill running, progress gradually as it will place strain on your muscles and can create significant muscle soreness in the quadriceps muscles in particular, due to eccentric muscle damage. A bout or two of downhill running can prevent further eccentric muscle damage for 4–6 weeks subsequently even if more downhill running is not carried out.

### Practising downhill running at a slower pace

If you are going to be running a race with significant downhill sections, it's worth including some downhill runs in your training, to accustom your muscles to the strain that they will be placed under in competitive conditions. When running down hill it's best to try not to fight the descent and to lean back and take smaller steps. Races can be won by those who are more adept than their competitors at running downhill and who are also conditioned to the eccentric forces involved and the break in rhythm placed by downhill sections.

## Sample uphill workouts

### Designed to develop power, speed and strength

- 10 x 40m sprints with 3 minutes' recovery between runs
- 3 x 4 x 60m sprints with 3 minutes between runs and 5 minutes between sets
- 2 x 5 x 80m sprints with 5 minutes between runs and 10 minutes between sets

### Designed to develop lactate threshold and tolerance

- 20 x 60m sprints at 90 per cent effort with walk-back recovery
- 3 x 6 x 80m runs at 80% per cent with walk-back recovery and 5 minutes between sets
- 2 x 10 x 60m sprints at 90 per cent with jog-back recovery

Note: Adjust the sessions according to your fitness, familiarity with fast running and the time in your training year.

## Sample downhill workouts

### Designed to develop sprint speed

Use a flat, dry grass slope of around 2 degrees and take as much recovery as you need between each run so that you can run flat out on each effort. You need to consider the drain that these sessions will have on your central nervous system (CNS); consequently, you need to be rested before them and not have an important race in the next few days following the workouts – it's best to take a rest day or to perform an easy recovery session the day after:

- 20m downhill sprint with 20m build-up speed approach x 4–6
- 2 x 30m downhill sprint, plus 4 x 50m on the flat sprints

### Designed to develop downhill race familiarity

Find some suitable terrain with hill climbs and descents and make a loop that lasts 5–10 minutes. Vary running fast and slower up and down the hills to create a different training effect.

Note: Although this session could, depending on its duration and intensity, develop aerobic or anaerobic fitness, the prime aim is to develop "hill" ability.

## Vibration training and running

Vibration training has become increasingly popular in the fitness and sports training world. Various manufacturers' machines are commonplace in gyms nationwide. However, whether they work or not – in terms of improving fitness or sports performance and recovery – is a matter of debate. This section provides an overview and takes a look at their general fitness and specific-to-running merits.

## History of vibration training

Vibration training has been around for 40 years, although its application for sport and fitness purposes has only recently begun to be more fully examined. It was developed in the Soviet Union in response to their space programme, specifically to keep a cosmonaut in space, in as best physical condition as possible for the longest period of time. The USSR held numerous endurance records in this respect.

Vibration training involves the use of machines that vibrate at frequencies, usually regulated to be between 30 and 50Hz. Most are platform-based – you stand on the plate and perform various exercises, some of which involve movement, such as single and double leg squats, while others utilise held positions, such as squatting and holding a half squat position.

**A typical vibration machine**

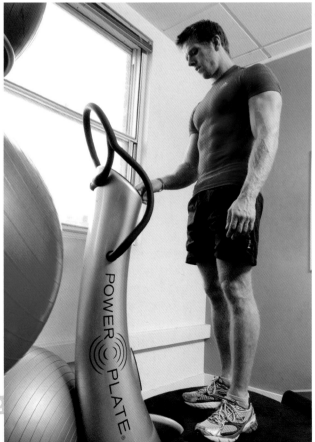

Other items of vibration equipment also exist, such as vibration dumbbells, and the concept has even been applied to breathing inspiration devices.

## Does vibration training work?

A peer research review (up to August 2005) by Swedish researchers found no real benefits of vibration training across various measures.[9] However, a similar review by New Zealanders did come up with slightly different findings – their research review took place a few years later.[10] However, their conclusions also do not make great reading for vibration equipment manufacturers: "Because whole-body vibration does not seem to be detrimental to performance when used in a controlled manner, it could provide an additional training stimulus for athletes." So there seems to be little vindication of whole body vibration training on its own merits.

I'd therefore recommend that if you as a runner want to use it, then it's probably best to do so as an adjunct to your training for strength and as a good way of boosting recovery after weights and running sessions. Vibration machines can be used when set at lower frequencies to aid recovery. They do this by stimulating muscular blood flow. Combining exercises performed on a relevant machine during/after a weights session could also be well worth trying. If in doubt about how to use a machine and/or what exercises to perform, consult an expert.

## Selected vibration machine exercises

For all the exercises set the machine up with your desired protocol (i.e. time, frequency and recovery). The higher the frequency, the greater the training effect in terms of muscle fibre activation. Use lower frequencies for recovery and when you're starting a programme of vibration training. Expect to feel a tingling, hot sensation – often in the calf muscles – when performing whole body vibration training. This is nothing to worry about and should quickly dissipate. If you are new to this type of training, always underestimate what you think you will be able to achieve.

# Strength

## Ex 8.56 Three-quarter squat on vibration machine

### Targets
This exercise targets the calf muscles, quadriceps, glutes and hamstrings.

### How to perform
Stand on the machine. Maintain a neutral spine position with head and chest lifted. Bend knees to between 130–160 degrees and extend your knees to return to the start position. Hold the machine's grip (if available).

### Variation
Hold the lowered position for a designated time.

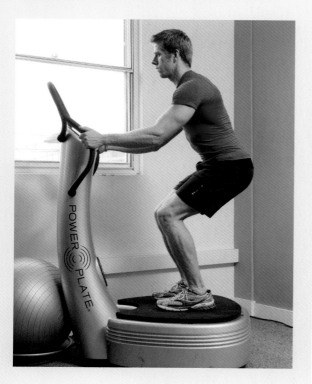

## Ex 8.57 Lunge on vibration machine

### Targets
This exercise targets the calf muscles, quadriceps, glutes and hamstrings.

### How to perform
Place one foot in the middle of the plate leaving the other on the ground. Keep your chest elevated and hands by your sides. Lower your body by bending your legs so that there is, or is near to, a 90-degree angle at both knee joints. Press back through your heel to return to the start position and repeat.

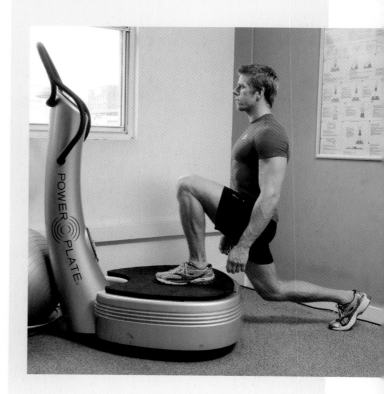

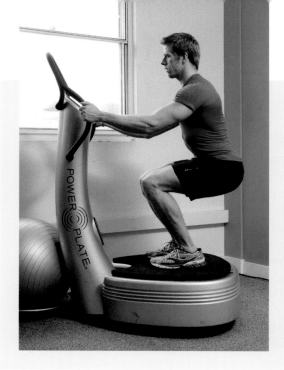

## Ex 8.58 Deep squat

### Targets
This exercise targets the calf muscles, quadriceps, glutes and hamstrings.

### How to perform
Stand on the machine. Maintain a neutral spine position with head and chest lifted. Bend your knees until your thighs are parallel (or near to) the ground position. Etend your knees to return to the start position and repeat. Hold the machine's grip (if available).

### Variation
Hold the lowered position for a designated time.

## Recovery

## Ex 8.59 Hamstring massage

### How to perform
From a seated position, place your legs on the machine so that your hamstrings are central to the plate. Support your body through your arms or place a similar height to the vibration machine such as a platform exercise class step in front of it, so that you can rest comfortably on the machine.

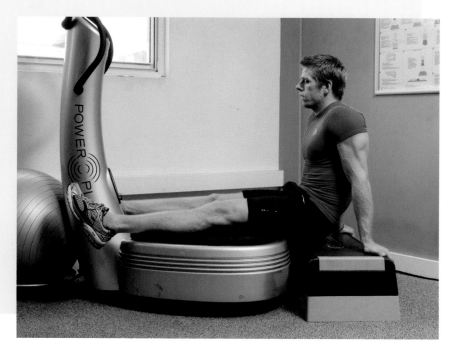

# Ex 8.60 Calf massage

**How to perform**
Assume a similar position to the exercise above, but this time place just your calf muscles on the plate.

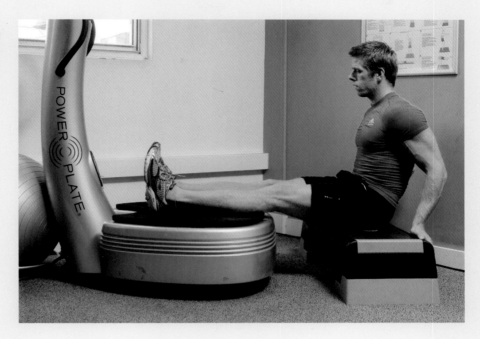

# References

1  Bell, G.J., Petersen, S.R., Quinney, A.H., Wenger, H.A. (1993), 'The effect of velocity-specific strength training on peak torque and anaerobic rowing power'. *Journal of Sports Sciences*, 1989; 7: 205-214

2  *Medicine and Science in Sports and Exercise*, 1994;26(5):575

3  Tanaka, H., Costill, D.L., Thomas, R., Fink, W.J., Widrick, J.J. (1993), 'Dry-land resistance training for competitive swimming'. *Medicine and Science in Sports and Exercise*, 25:952-959

4  Paavolainen, L., Hakkinen, K., Rusko, H. (1991), 'Effects of explosive type strength training on physical performance characteristics in cross-country skiers'. *European Journal of Applied Physiology*, 62:251-255.

5  'Theory and practice of strength development'. In Dick, F. *Sports Training Principles* 4th edn. (A & C Black, 2002):238

6  Shepard, R.J. (1978), 'Aerobic vs Anaerobic Training for success in various athletic events', *Canadian Journal of Applied Sport Sciences, 3*, 9-15

7  Spoorer (2003), 'Effects of aerobic exercise on strength performance following various periods of recovery'. *Journal of Strength & Conditioning Research*, Nov17(4):638-644

8  'Sequencing of endurance and high velocity training', *Canadian Journal of Applied Sport Science*, 1988;13(4):214-19

9  *Scandinavian Journal of Medicine & Science in Sports*, 2007 Feb; 17(1):12-7

10  *Journal of Strength & Conditioning Research*, 2009 Mar; 23(2):593-603

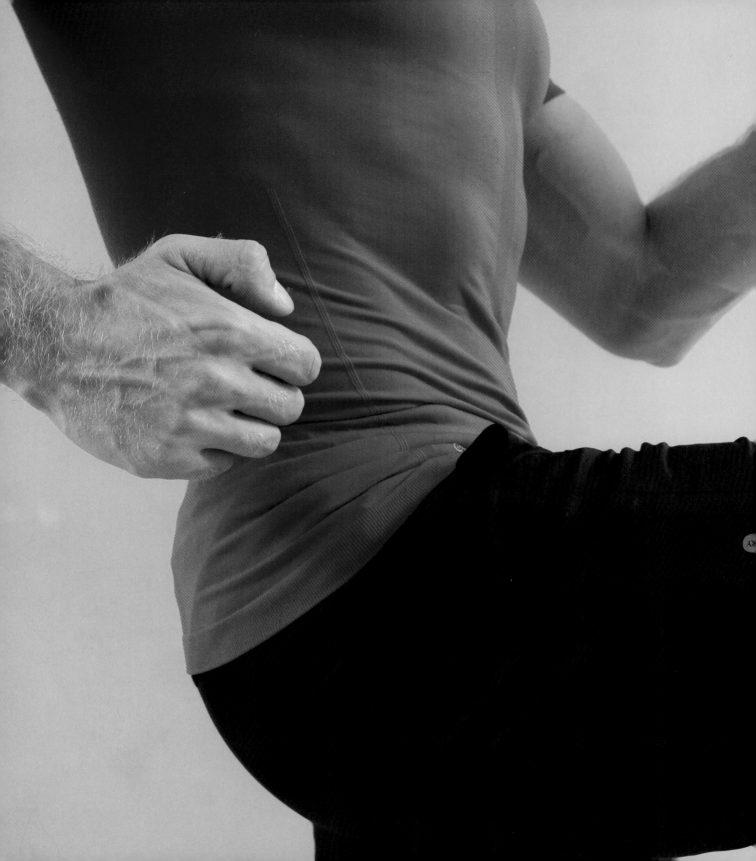

# 9

# core strength for runners

Your core is crucial for stronger running – it transmits the forces generated by your limbs and if not suitably conditioned will reduce your running efficiency. A weak core will also increase your chances of injury, in particular in the lower back and other body parts.

There are lots of ways to train your core. You'll undoubtedly be familiar with exercises such as sit-ups and crunches. Although these are very valuable exercises, they are perhaps slightly less effective compared to more static (isometric) "held" exercises, such as the plank and its variations, which target the deeper abdominal muscles, such as the transversus obliques and erector spinae back muscles. Crunches and other similar flexion/extension exercises, predominantly target the larger "surface" muscle, the rectus abdominis ("six-pack" muscle), whereas the held exercises engage the deeper core muscles as well.

Having said that, it is also important to include rotational movements in your core training to develop the muscles that combat the twisting forces that you'll be subjected to when running. And you can also train your core very dynamically, through the use of Powerbags and medicine balls. These exercises require

your core to anchor transmit the power generated by your limbs and control the additional load. In this chapter you'll find examples of all these types of core exercises and numerous workout examples. Your core training for running should incorporate all variations where possible.

## Key core muscles

### Front
**Rectus abdominis**
The rectus abdominis is the long slab of muscle that runs down the front of your core and is responsible for lifting and pulling it forwards and controlling its path backwards. It's also the muscle that will give those lucky few a six-pack. I say "lucky few" as genetics as well as a very demanding training programme are responsible for creating those most desirable peaks and valleys across your stomach. However, training for a "cosmetic" six-pack should be of secondary importance to you as a runner – rather you should focus on developing core muscles whose function it is to boost your running performance. If in the process you

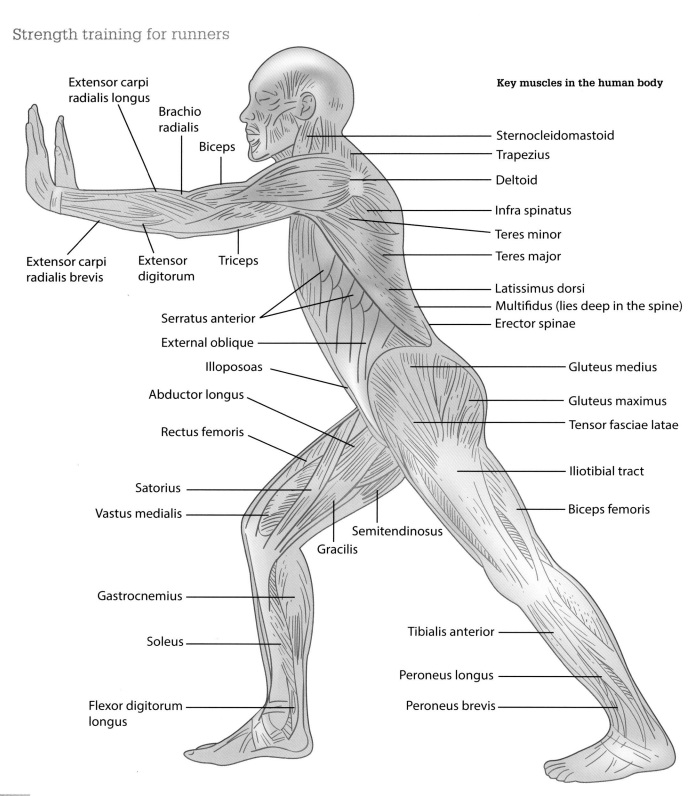

Extensor carpi
radialis longus

Brachio
radialis

Biceps

Extensor carpi
radialis brevis

Extensor
digitorum

Triceps

Key muscles in the human body

Sternocleidomastoid

Trapezius

Deltoid

Infra spinatus

Teres minor

Teres major

Latissimus dorsi

Multifidus (lies deep in the spine)

Erector spinae

Serratus anterior

External oblique

Illoposoas

Abductor longus

Rectus femoris

Satorius

Vastus medialis

Gluteus medius

Gluteus maximus

Tensor fasciae latae

Iliotibial tract

Biceps femoris

Semitendinosus

Gracilis

Gastrocnemius

Soleus

Tibialis anterior

Peroneus longus

Flexor digitorum
longus

Peroneus brevis

develop a great set of visually appealing abs then that's a bonus!

The rectus abdominis is one large muscle. Certain specific exercises can, however, emphasise parts of it, for example, the lower region.

## Internal and external obliques

These muscles facilitate twisting and turning movements and also support the spine. The internal and external obliques are trained with exercises, such as alternate knee to elbow crunches ("chinnies", see exercise 8.11, page 102). These muscles are important in the battle against the rotational forces that are generated by running. If you have obliques that are under trained, then it's likely that you will not be able to control these forces, which are produced by your legs and arms, particularly when running at faster paces and especially when sprinting. Twisting trunk movements dissipate and waste force from where it is needed – in a straight line to push you forward.

## Transversus abdominis

These deep lying core muscles (they reside below the obliques) work in harmony with the other abdominal and spinal muscles to stabilise the spine and contribute to posture.

## Sides

### Quadratus lumborum

The quadratus lumborum is located to the sides of the torso and has an inner and outer portion. The inner portion connects directly to the spine and contributes

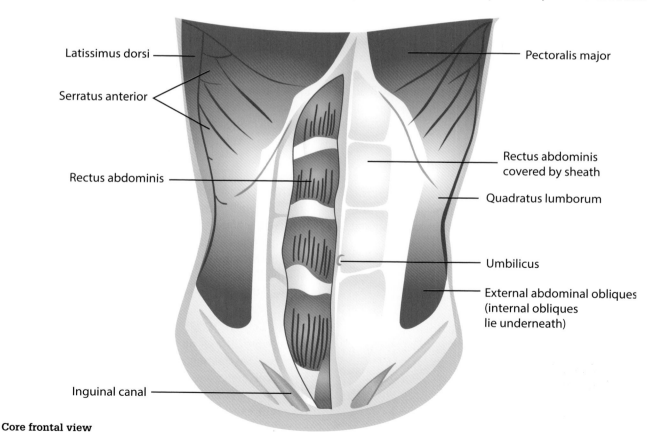

Latissimus dorsi

Serratus anterior

Rectus abdominis

Inguinal canal

Pectoralis major

Rectus abdominis covered by sheath

Quadratus lumborum

Umbilicus

External abdominal obliques (internal obliques lie underneath)

**Core frontal view**

to stability. Back pain is often the result of a tight outer portion of this muscle.

## Back
### Multifidus
These muscles work with the abdominals to hold the body upright. They attach to single vertebrae and cover a single area of the spine. The multifidus' key movement contribution is in stiffening the spine.

### Erector spinae
These muscles also control posture. They also assist with lowering torso movements, such as bending forwards. They are known as "global" muscles and can be viewed as two pillars on either side of the spinal column. When the back is injured these muscles can often take a while to be "re-trained" to perform the function they were designed to. They are relatively lazy muscles and will "adopt bad habits", which can result in poor posture. The erector spinae can become lazy as we age and as we slump at computers and spend so much of our time sitting. Poor general posture can lead to problems when running in terms of maintenance of good technique and potential injury.

### The hips
The iliopsoas, which is in reality two muscles, the psoas and the iliacus, are involved in core training. The former attaches to the spine and is therefore important for core stability and the latter contributes to abdominal

exercises, such as the sit-up, when the trunk is pulled towards the legs.

### Gluteus medius
The gluteus medius is situated on the upper sides of the hips and runs into the small of the back. These muscles are important a) for injury avoidance and b) for good running technique. When trained, they contribute to a core that optimises linear transference of force and reduces twisting movement when running.

## How may reps and sets?
I have not provided reps and sets for the core exercises described in this section. If you perform any of the selected exercises as part of a weights or circuit training session, you can use the protocols provided for the sample workouts earlier in this chapter. You can also include them as a training unit in separate workouts – perhaps selecting two to three to perform. And you can even include them in your warm-up. Whichever way you include your core exercises in your training you must always strive to complete them with perfect form, in order to fully recruit your core muscles over the optimum range of movement for the exercise. Failure to do so can result in compromised training adaptation.

## A note on speed of movement
For the moving (isotonic) exercises that involve eccentric and concentric muscular actions, try to complete them to a steady "one count" lifting phase and "two count" lowering phase, where appropriate. It's important that you control gravity when lowering your trunk, as this will work your core muscles eccentrically and create greater all-round strength development.

## Progressions
If you have little or no training experience of dynamic core exercise training, such as those involving medicine ball throwing, then spend time developing a sound base of core strength first using the other isotonic and isometric exercises.

> ### Great running core strength exercises
> Core exercises can be found elsewhere in this book, for example as part of pre-conditioning and weight training workouts (see page 95). You'll find explanations for exercises such as the plank and alternate elbow to knee sit-ups in these sections.

# Isometric exercises for the core

## Ex 9.1 Side plank with rotation

### Targets
This exercise targets the obliques and the shoulders.

### How to perform
Lie on your side and lift your body so that your supporting elbow is below your shoulder and your lower arm is facing forwards. Stack your feet and hips over one another. There should be a straight line running from your top ear, through your shoulder, hip, knee and ankle. Reach up with your free arm so that it is at right angles to the ground – this is the start position. Hold for a two-count and then take that arm's hand under your body, rotating your torso as you do so – your hand should end up pointing behind you and you should be able to look under your body. Pause and take the arm back to the start position. Complete your designated number of repetitions and repeat on the other side

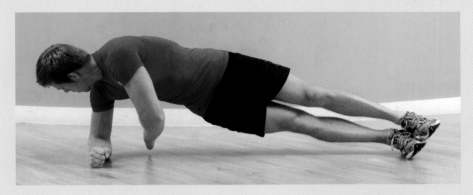

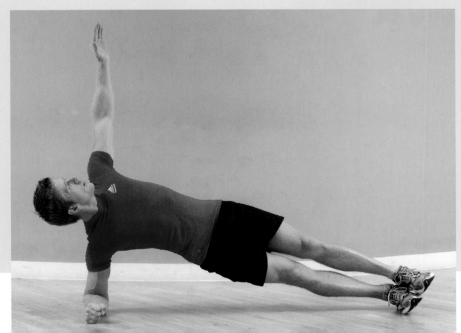

## Ex 9.2 Arms extended plank

**Targets**
This exercise targets the obliques, erector spinae, rectus abdominus, bottom, shoulders and quadriceps.

**How to perform**
Assume a press-up type position with arms extended as per image. Brace your core to hold this position for a designated period of time and then swap legs. Aim to keep as square as you can throughout the exercise and control your breathing.

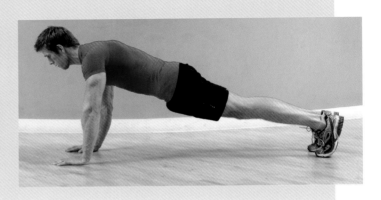

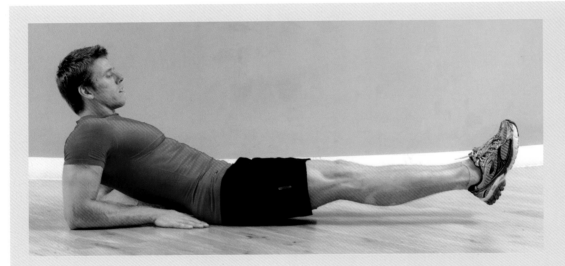

## Ex 9.3 Leg lifts

**Targets**
This exercise targets the rectus abdominus, erector spinae, hip flexors and shoulders.

**How to perform**
Lie on your back and lift your trunk slightly while supporting your torso on your elbows. Lift your legs 30–50cm from the floor and hold the position for a designated time span. Do not attempt to lift your legs any higher as this can place strain on the muscles of the lower back. Lower under control.

**Progression**
Hold a medicine ball between your feet.

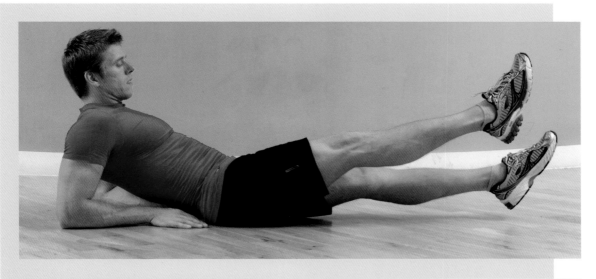

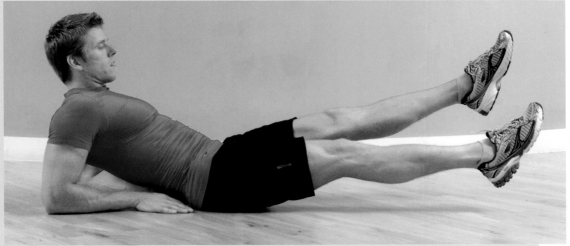

# Ex 9.4 Flutter kicks

**Targets**
This exercise targets the rectus abdominus and hip flexors.

**How to perform**
Assume the same starting position as for exercise 9.3, however, this time, on elevating your legs, scissor them through a short range of movement, while keeping your legs extended. Try counting slowly "one-two", "one-two", in time with each left and right leg movement.

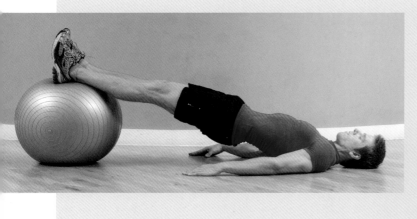

## Ex 9.5 Swiss ball glute bridge

### Targets
This exercise targets the erector spinae, abdominals, obliques, hamstrings and bottom.

### How to perform
Sit facing the Swiss ball, lie back, extend your legs and place your heels on the top of the ball about hip-width apart. Extend your arms by your sides. Push into the ball with your heels and lift your hips. Maintain a straight line through your heels to your upper back. Hold for a designated period and lower under control.

## Ex 9.6 Swiss ball plank

### Targets
This exercise targets the rectus abdominus.

### How to perform
Place your forearms on the top of the Swiss ball and walk your feet back so that you are in a plank position. As with all plank variations, focus on keeping your body in correct alignment. The instability of the Swiss ball will add to the muscular recruitment of the exercise, as you have to work that little bit harder to hold yourself still.

### Variation
The exercise can also be performed in reverse with your shins on the ball and hands on the ground (see Ex 9.8, image 1).

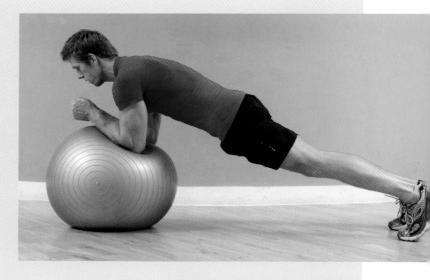

### Running training tip
Include a set of abdominal exercises in your warm-up. This is a time-effective way of making sure that you develop and maintain core strength across your training.

## Isotonic exercises

### Ex 9.7 Lying bent leg torso twists

**Targets**
This exercise targets the obliques and glute medius.

**How to perform**
Lie on your back with your hands outstretched and backs of hands on the ground in a crucifix-type position. Bring your legs in towards your torso, bending them at the knees. With your thighs at right angles to the ground, rotate your legs slowly to one side. Stop the movement a couple of centimetres from the floor and then take your legs over to the other side. Keep your shoulders down at all times. As you exercise confidence and strength develops and you can increase the speed of the exercise.

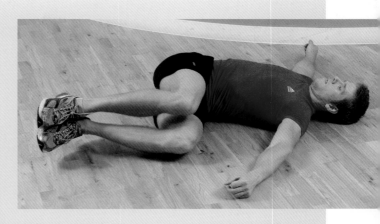

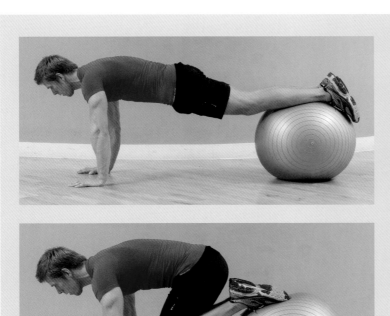

### Ex 9.8 Swiss ball jackknife

**Targets**
This exercise targets the rectus abdominus and hip flexors.

**How to perform**
Get into a press-up position with your hands on the floor and your shins resting on the Swiss ball. Your body should be perfectly horizontal. Contract your abs, drive your hips up towards the ceiling and pull your knees in towards your chest. Extend your legs to push the ball away and return to the starting position.

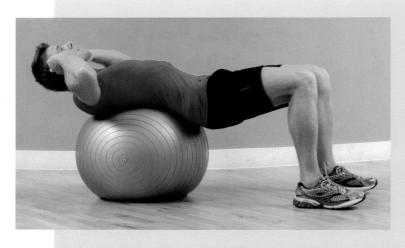

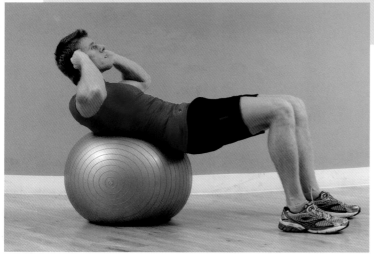

### Ex 9.9 Swiss ball crunch

**Targets**
This exercise targets the rectus abdominus.

**How to perform**
Sit on the Swiss ball and lie on it so that it sits in the natural curve of your lower back. Position your fingers by your temples and keep your elbows out. Wrap your back around the ball. Your head should be level or slightly below your hips. Exhale and curl your shoulders off the ball. Focus on crunching your abdominals as opposed to sitting up from your hips. Pause and then return to the starting position.

## Swiss balls

Swiss balls are highly versatile and useful pieces of kit. They provide a base for a multitude of exercises, core and otherwise. The performance of, for example, a plank on a Swiss ball requires greater core control and promotes increased muscle recruitment, compared to performing the exercise without one. This results from your muscles having to work harder due to the instability of the ball.

### Swiss ball guide to sizes

| Your height (cm) | Ball size (cm) |
| --- | --- |
| 188+ | Large: 75cm |
| 168–188+ | Medium: 65cm |
| 152–168+ | Small: 55cm |

Go for an anti-burst ball!

## Ex 9.10 Swiss ball Russian twist

### Targets

This exercise targets the obliques, rectus abdominus and glutes.

### How to perform

Sit on the ball and walk your feet away until the ball is behind your shoulders. Your thighs should be parallel to the floor, your shins vertical and feet flat on the floor. Extend your arms over your chest and clasp your hands together. Rotate your upper body from side to side, lifting one shoulder off the ball at a time, all the while keeping your hips level.

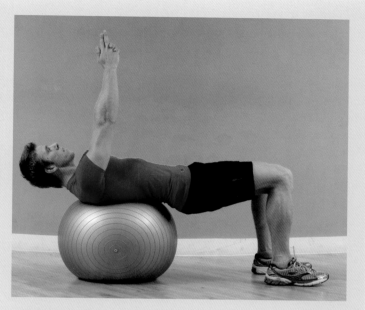

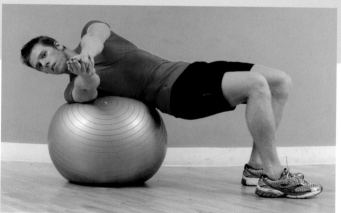

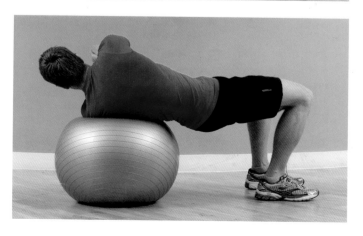

167

## What's a plyometric action?

Muscles can exert more power when an eccentric action precedes a concentric one. The eccentric action is akin to an elastic band being stretched – the muscle lengthens under load – while the concentric, muscle-shortening-under-load action is akin to what happens when the elastic band is released. In the split second of recoil immense amounts of energy are released. Plyometric training is a great way to develop explosive power and is a mainstay of sports training – yet most runners don't use it for their core.

## Why plyometrically train your core for running?

Plyometric core exercises, if performed sensibly and by the suitably conditioned, will add another dimension to your "running core". The fact that you are able to handle explosive movements through this region will further strengthen and make for even more injury-resilient running. Additionally, the movements require the co-ordination of leg and arm actions, which is a running requirement. Your whole body has to work synergistically and not with a particular part in isolation, which makes for a very sports-specific outcome.

## Plyometric exercises for the core: Medicine ball exercises

### Ex 9.11 Medicine ball sideways throw against wall

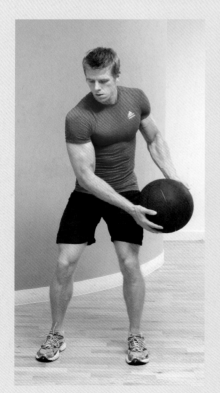

**Targets**
This exercise targets the obliques, chest, shoulders, legs and hips.

**How to perform**
Assume a two-footed side-on stance facing a wall (left foot closest to wall) and back from it. Hold the medicine ball in two hands at arm's length and rotate first to the right, turning through your hips and ankles. Then dynamically rotate back towards the wall and throw the medicine ball. Catch the rebound. Complete a designated number of repetitions and then change your foot stance and throw to the other side.

**Variations**
See exercise 8.55, page 147 for the medicine ball chest pass against a wall.

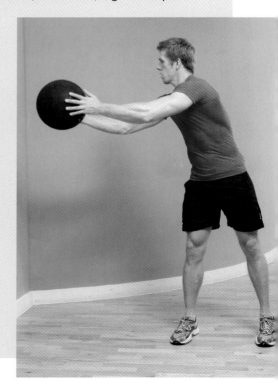

# Ex 9.12 Medicine ball sit-up and throw

## Targets
This exercise targets the rectus abdominus, chest, shoulders.

## How to perform
You'll need a training partner to get the most out of this exercise (although you can throw the ball against a wall and collect the rebound). Take hold of a medicine ball and assume a sit-up position, with feet flat on the floor and knees bent to an angle of 90 degrees. Hold the medicine ball on your chest with your hands to the sides of it. Lower your back towards the floor then, using your abdominal muscles, pull your trunk forwards dynamically. Near the top of the movement throw the ball to your partner (or against the wall) using a chest pass action, i.e. push your arms dynamically away from you to throw the ball. Your partner should catch the ball and toss it back just as you are sitting back, ready to perform your next rep. Aim to "catch and move forwards to throw" as quickly as possible.

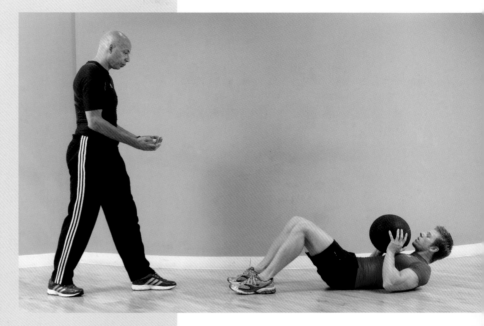

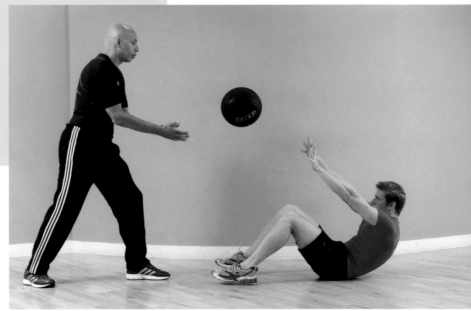

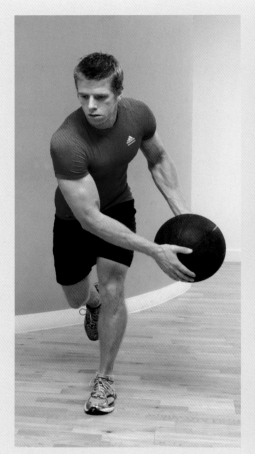 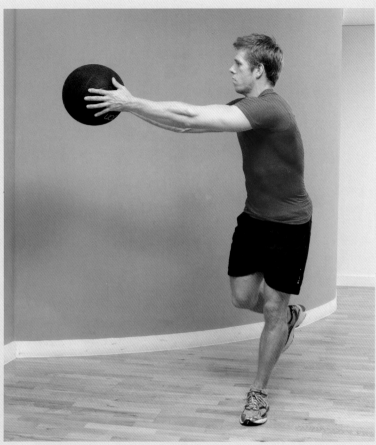

## Ex 9.13 Single leg, medicine ball twist, throw and catch

### Targets

This exercise targets the core (obliques in particular), glute medius, legs and arms. Having to combat the transverse forces that run through your core (and body) when making the throw and the catch will develop reactive and stabilising core strength. By training your glute medius in particular (outer hips) you will find that your running stability improves as you develop strength and balance in a further, very-important-to-running body part.

### How to perform

Ideally you'll need a training partner to perform this exercise (although you can throw the ball against a wall). Stand on one leg, tucking the heel of your other leg up towards your bottom. Hold the medicine ball at arm's length in front of you and parallel to the ground. Your partner should stand to the opposite side to the ball and about a metre away. Throw the ball to your partner (or against the wall), who then catches it and throws it back to you. Catch the ball and rotate away from the wall with the ball held at arm's length and make a further throw.

## Isometric/more slowly performed core exercises

The descriptions that follow focus on the use of medicine balls, dumbbells and ViPRs. Dumbbells make for a great running strength training piece of kit. They can be used singularly or in pairs and allow for relative flexibility in use and movement. They're also great for addressing balance and co-ordination.

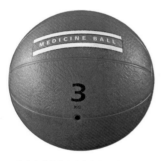

### Dynamic running core training – using medicine balls, dumbbells and ViPRs

This equipment enables a myriad of core (and other body part) exercises to be performed. You can use them to add resistance to your training like "hard" weights, such as barbells and kettlebells, but their obvious beauty is their relative portability. This makes them ideal for dynamic exercises – you can jump with them, throw them and catch them.

Like Swiss balls, medicine balls are multiple-use pieces of kit that can easily be kept at home. Use them as resistance for all manner of exercises, not just your core. Go for a ball that weighs 3kg, 4kg or 5kg, depending on your strength and experience.

ViPRs can be found in many gyms up and down the country. They are made from rubber and have numerous grips and holds. This enables them to be lifted, rotated and thrown in numerous ways.

## Ex 9.14 Resisted Medicine ball crunch

### Targets

This exercise targets the rectus abdominus and shoulders, using a held isometric muscular action.

### How to perform

Assume a sit-up position. Your heels should be on the floor and knees bent to an angle of 90 degrees. Take hold of a medicine ball and hold it at arm's length, allowing it to drop back over your wrists. Lean very slightly backwards and hold this contracted position for 10 seconds.

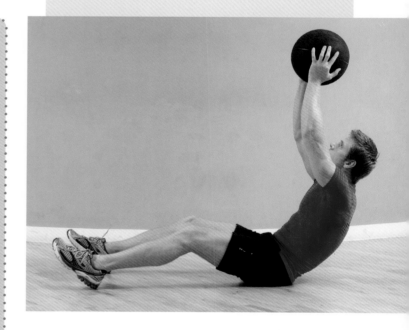

## Ex 9.15 Medicine ball twists

### Targets
This exercise targets the obliques. This is a great exercise for developing rotational core strength that will assist you in maintaining a strong running posture.

### How to perform
Stand with your feet shoulder-width apart and hug a medicine ball to your chest. Rotate from left to right at a moderate tempo.

### Progression
Hold a medicine ball at arm's length and rotate your trunk as described – this is a more advanced exercise and will require greater stabilisation work on the part of the core and in particular the upper back. The exercise will also strengthen your shoulders.

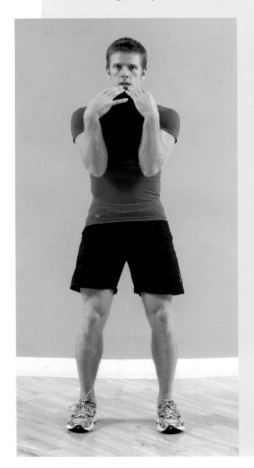
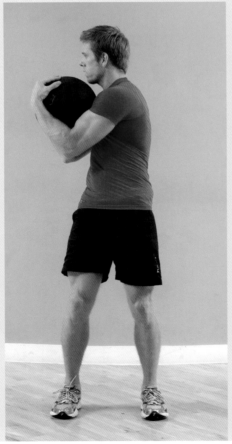
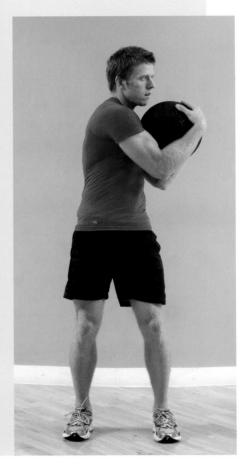

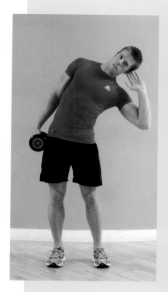
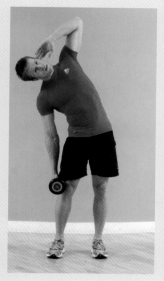

## Ex 9.16 Dumbbell side bend

### Targets
This exercise targets the obliques. Side bends are a simple, but very effective way to target these muscles.

### How to perform
Stand with your feet shoulder-width apart holding a dumbbell at arm's length. Let it hang down by the side of one leg. Fold your other arm so that your hand is close to your ear and its upper arm parallel to the ground. Lean slowly sideways allowing the dumbbell to slide down your leg. Don't let the weight swing and don't lean forwards or backwards from your hips. Return to upright, by contracting the obliques on the opposite side to the dumbbell.

## Ex 9.17 ViPR dynamic walking figure of eight

### Targets
This exercise targets the obliques, upper back, shoulders, legs and will assist postural control and balance.

### How to perform
Stand with your feet shoulder-width apart. Hold the ViPR by its grips in front of you at near to arm's length. Take a step forward into a lunge with your left leg, at the same time shovelling the ViPR up and over into an arc, so it crosses your body. Your top hand should rise to about shoulder height. Control the descent – this is tough and will require you to maintain your balance. The ViPR should end

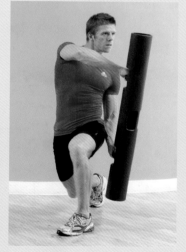
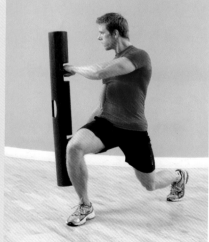

up outside the thigh of your forward leg. Step into another lunge with your other leg and reverse the swing of the ViPR. Change your starting position and grip after each rep (two lunges) or after completing a designated number of repetitions.

## Wall bars/high bar exercises

Wall bars, a chinning bar or a gymnastics high bar make for great tools to train your abdominals and in particular the lower region of the rectus abdominus and the hip flexors. In terms of being beneficial to running, these exercises will strengthen the muscles that lift and lower your knees, which will benefit faster running where you have to drive your thighs powerfully up and forwards. They will also teach you postural control and help you to develop greater core awareness as, rather like suspended body weight training (see page 176), you'll not be anchored to the ground when performing the exercises and will therefore have to combat rotation and swaying momentum.

Those new to this type of training should progress slowly over time – as these exercises require considerable postural control and core strength.

### Ex 9.18 Hang and double bent knee leg lift

**Targets**
This exercise targets the rectus abdominus and hip flexors.

**How to perform**
Hang from the wall bars at arm's length, so that your feet are off the floor. Keeping your feet close together, lift your thighs to parallel to the ground – your lower legs should be at right angles to your thighs. Pause and extend your legs under control back to the start position. Don't use momentum to swing your legs up. You need to brace your core and fix yourself in position.

If using a high bar, then the intensity of the exercise is increased as you have to work that much harder to control your movements and keep any swaying to a minimum as there is no support behind you (as below).

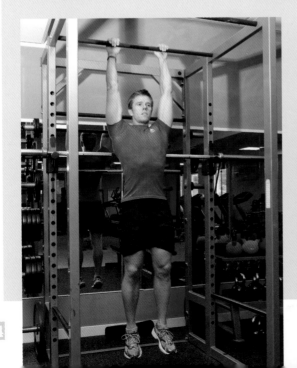 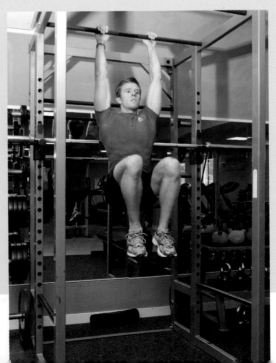

## Ex 9.19 Hang and straight leg lift

### Targets
This exercise targets the rectus abdominus and hip flexors.

### How to perform
Hang from the wall bars at arm's length, so that your feet are off the floor. Keeping your feet close together, lift your legs so that they rise to a position parallel to the ground. Pause and lower your legs under control back to the start position. This is a demanding exercise and you must keep your back pressed into the wall bars. If using a high bar then, as exercise 9.18, the intensity is significantly increased.

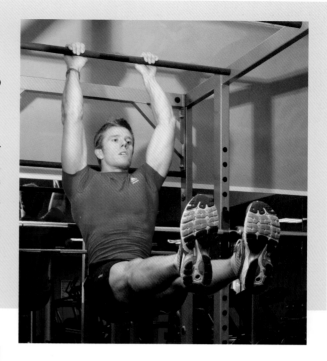

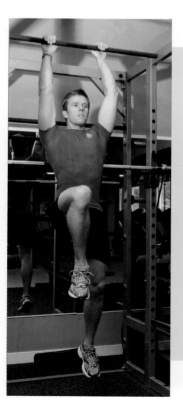

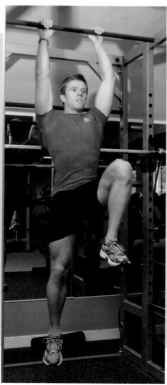

## Ex 9.20 Hang and alternate single leg lift

### Targets
This exercise targets the rectus abdominus and hip flexors.

### How to perform
Hang from the wall bars at arm's length, so that your feet are off the floor. Keeping one leg extended, lift the other so that its thigh reaches a position parallel to the floor. Pause lower and repeat with the other leg.

### Ex 9.21 Hang and straight leg lift with hold

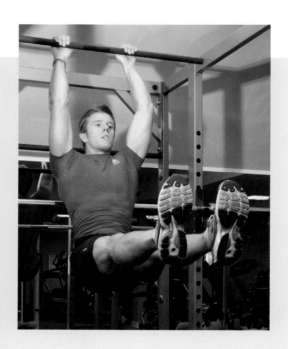

**Targets**
This exercise targets the rectus abdominus and hip flexors (will emphasise the latter during the hold in particular).

**How to perform**
Hang from the wall bars at arm's length, so that your feet are off the floor. Keeping your feet close together, lift your legs so that they rise to a position parallel to the ground. At the top of the movement hold your legs in position for a 5-second count. Lower your legs under control back to the start position. This again is a very demanding exercise – it should only be performed by the very well and specifically conditioned.

## Suspended body weight training for the core

Suspension Training® systems are a great, relatively new way to train your core (and other muscles). The exercises require you to control your body weight while you are suspended to some degree or another. This requires balance, greater postural control, body awareness and proprioception (see pages 12–13).

### Ex 9.22 Roll-out

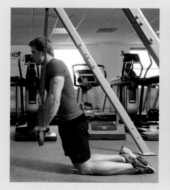
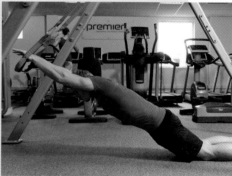

**Targets**
This exercise targets the rectus abdominus and shoulders.

**How to perform**
Kneel with your back to the anchor point and the device running over your shoulders. Grasp a handle in each hand. From this position, push the handles away from you and lower your upper body towards the floor. Aim to fully extend your arms so that your body is virtually parallel to it, although you should only lean as far as is comfortable. Hold the end position for 1–2 seconds and then use your core muscles to pull you back upright. Do not allow your lower back to arch as this can lead to injury. If you feel this exercise in your lower back, reduce your range of movement or shorten the straps.

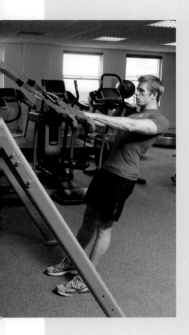

## Ex 9.23 Back extension

### Targets
This exercise targets the erector spinae, rear shoulders, upper back and glutes.

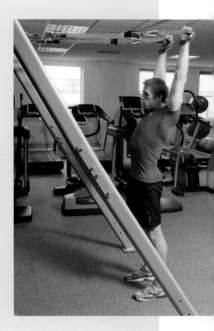

### How to perform
Stand facing the anchor point and hold a handle in each hand. With your arms straight and feet together, lean back slightly so your weight is supported on your extended arms. Arch your back slightly, push your hips forwards and raise your arms above your head. Use the muscles on the rear of your body to lift you into an upright position. Return to the starting position and repeat.

To reduce the intensity of the exercise you can use a split stance and use your rear leg to assist your arms. Remember: this is a core exercise so focus on a strong hip and back extension.

## Ex 9.24 Side hip lift

### Targets
This exercise targets the obliques, rectus abdominus, erector spinae.

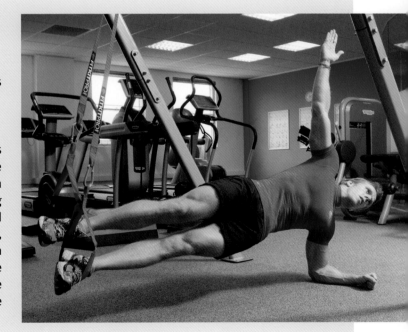

### How to perform
Sit down and place both feet in the device's handles. Your feet should be about 15cm off the floor. Roll onto your side and rest your weight on your lower-most arm, as though you are performing side planks. Make sure your hips are squared (stacked on top of each other). From this position, lower your bottom hip to touch the floor and then lift your hips as high as you can. Repeat for the designated number of repetitions and then change sides. To aid your balance you can place your free hand on the floor in front of your waist.

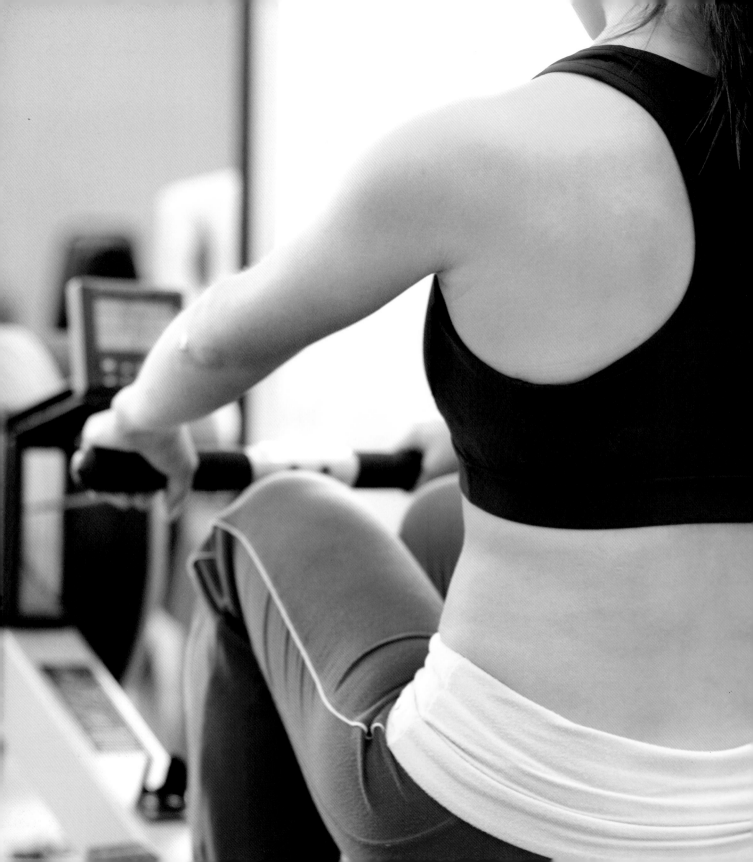

# 10 cross-training for stronger running

Cross-training involves including non-running based training methods into your training to enhance your running. In this way all forms of training, such as weights, circuit training and plyometrics, qualify as cross-training, in that they "break" up the demands placed on the body by "just" running and can enhance performance. For the purposes of this chapter we'll focus on the cardiovascular (CV) elements that can usefully be added to an overall training programme and contribute towards making you a faster runner.

## Why cross-train?

- Cross-training can prevent run-training boredom and provide mental stimulation.
- Cross-training can reduce overuse injuries by varying and spreading the training load and impact forces across the body and its different muscles.
- Cross-training can address running induced muscular imbalances.
- Cross-training can boost recovery after tough sessions and reduce the overall loading placed on the body, if implemented systematically into a progressive training plan.
- Cross-training can at the least maintain running condition, and in some cases enhance it.
- Cross-training can enhance joint mobility.
- Repeated running requires a relatively limited range of movement – with "more and more" miles the range of movement around a joint, such as the knee, can decrease as muscles, tendons and ligaments shorten. The hamstrings and calf muscles are particularly prone to this happening. Cross-training can reduce the chances of this.
- Cross-training can contribute to maintaining desired body fat levels. A cross-training activity can create an additional calorie burn. Reducing body fat safely can enhance performance. For example, a 70kg runner who reduces their body fat by 1.5kg could take around 2 minutes off their 10k time.
- Cross-training can boost mental toughness. It's often argued that the best endurance runners are those with superior mental toughness – they are better prepared for success when racing (they have greater self-belief, for example) and are

better able to cope with difficult patches when racing. In short, they have better mental toughness. Intense non-running based CV workouts can help develop this.

- Cross-training can allow for a more intense training workload across a training period. Most sub-elite level, training mature marathon runners really only directly benefit from one to two runs a week – traditionally the long weekend run. Their other shorter efforts performed during the week tend to have more of a maintenance effect on fitness. Too many hard running workouts create stress on the musculoskeletal system and can potentially lead to injury. However, a strategically placed hard cycle or indoor rowing session, for example, could create similar CV effects, but without the same stress on the body.

## Cycling and running

Cycling is a great way to develop leg power, aerobic and anaerobic endurance. Although the range of movement required for cycling is much more limited compared to running, this is in part offset by the fact that it is weight bearing and produces little impact on the body.

Researchers from the University of Texas reviewed existing studies on the transfer of cross-training effects to VO2max, between cycling, running and swimming.[1] As we have seen, VO2max refers to the maximum amount of oxygen the body can process (measured either in litres per minute or in millilitres per minute per kilo of body weight). They determined that there is a transfer of training effects in terms of VO2max from one training method to another. More specifically they noted that running had the greatest positive transference and swimming the least, with cycling ranked in the middle.

One piece of specific field research considered the value of cycling as a training means between the cross-country and track season for female distances runners.[2] Specifically, the researchers wanted to find our whether substituting 50 per cent of running training volume with cycling could maintain 3000m track race performance and VO2max during a five-week recuperative phase at the end of the cross-country season. The 11 runners in the study formed two groups:

1. A run-only group
2. A run and cycle training group, which performed the two different activities on different days

Both groups trained at 75–85 per cent of maximum heart rate (MHR). Training volumes were similar to the competitive season, except, as noted, cycling made up 50 per cent of the volume of the run and cycle group. At the end of the five-week period the team discovered that 3000m race times were on average 9 seconds, or 1.4 per cent slower in the run-only group, and 22 seconds, or 3.4% slower, in the run and cycle group. Equally important, if not more so for the value of cross-training, was the fact that the VO2max of both groups remained the same.

The implications of this research go beyond recommending cycling as a valuable means for cross-training at the transition between running seasons, as the findings indicate that cycling can contribute toward running performance on an all-year round basis. This is because:

- cycling may enable the runner's body more time to recover from tough training/competitive training phases and improve future injury resilience; and

- from a mental perspective, the involvement of a different training method (cycling) may help to "rejuvenate" the mental approach of endurance athletes and ultimately boost performance.

On the face of the available evidence, using cycling as a means to improve/maintain your running endurance seems worth experimenting with. Introducing the activity in a way similar to that used in the 3000m running study shown above could be a useful starting point, i.e. at a transition phase in training (for example, at the beginning of a recovery period) and with a 1:1 (i.e. "like for like" in terms of intensity) ratio of cycling and running. As a rough guide, cycle distances should be increased threefold in comparison to running distances in order to achieve a similar cardiovascular training effect. Heart rate levels should be the same in order to maintain similar intensity.

### Cycling and eccentric muscle damage

Running guru Dr Tim Noakes believes that cycling can be of further benefit to endurance runners, and particularly those post 35 years of age and those involved in the marathon and ultra-distance events.[3] This, he argues, is because of cycling's role in injury prevention and in particular the increasing inability of the legs to withstand prolonged eccentric muscular damage, which he sees as an inevitable consequence of years of distance running. Noakes believes that this damage will slow down even the most circumspect runners with age. As we have already seen, an eccentric muscular action occurs when a muscle lengthens under load. This happens, for example, in the quadriceps muscles every time they absorb the impact on foot strike – the load on the body will at minimum be three times greater than the runner's body weight. The quadriceps muscles are placed under even greater eccentric strain during downhill running (a condition likely to induce considerable muscle soreness when performed for the first time or after a prolonged break).

In short, Noakes believes that cycling can offer respite from eccentric muscular damage, potentially

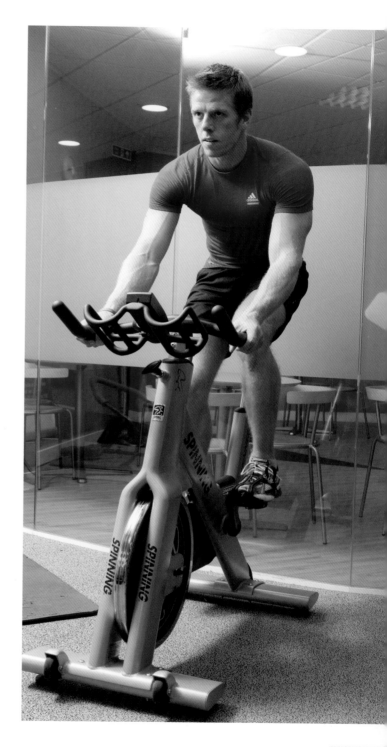

prolonging marathon and ultra-marathon endurance and older athletes' running careers (see chapter 11 for a more detailed consideration of the latter). Noakes believes that such an approach can even enhance performance and he cites triathlon as a case in point, where some of the world's very best triathletes have achieved prodigious endurance running performances despite relatively modest running training. He provides the following explanations:

- Cycling can produce the same metabolic stress on the body without the same loading stresses on the muscles and the skeleton (particularly, eccentric running muscle damage, as noted previously).
- Cycling may also help to "programme" the brain to withstand the mental aspect of completing an activity, such as an Ironman triathlon, that could last 10 hours or more. To bolster this argument he cites the case of one of the world's greatest-ever triathletes, Mark Allen, who he observed only gained Hawaiian Ironman success after he performed specifically intense cycling workouts.

## Boxing-based circuit training, running and calorific expenditure

Many runners – particularly those training for recreational purposes and improved health – may have done boxing-based workouts (or similar exercise class formats) as part of a cross-training/fitness routine, or might be thinking of doing so. So how physiologically effective are these types of exercise as a form of cross-training and can they provide sport-specific benefits for running?

Boxing circuit classes typically take 45–60 minutes to complete and involve skipping, circuit exercises for the whole body (such as press-ups and crunches) and, occasionally (for more advanced trainers), bag or pad

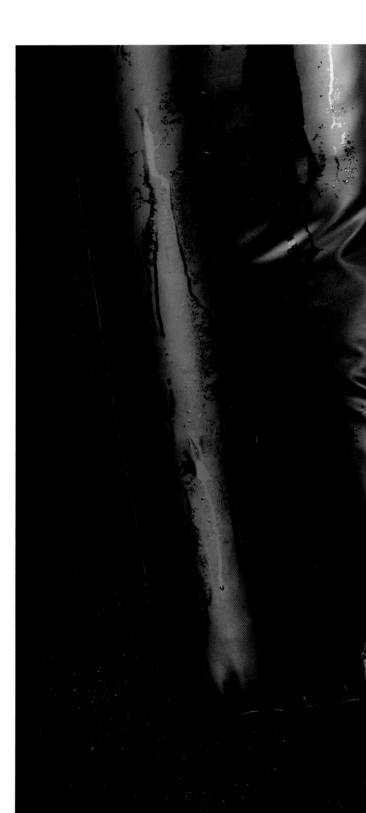

Boxing-based fitness classes can
boost your running strength

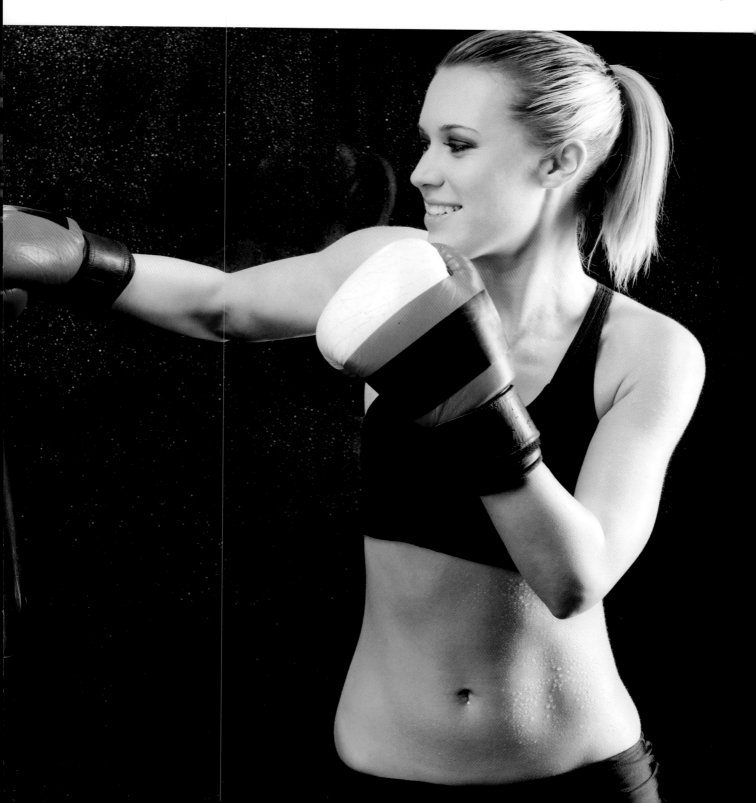

work and shadow boxing. Recoveries are kept to a minimum and the workouts can be very tough. They predominantly tax the start-stop anaerobic energy system.

Researchers compared boxing-based circuits to treadmill running to determine energy expenditure.[1] Eight men with boxing-based class workout experience took part in the study, and they were divided into three class types:

1  An hour's boxing-based workout in a laboratory
2  An hour's boxing-based workout in a gym
3  An incremental run on a treadmill

In the lab and gym, the men burned 671 and 599 calories respectively. Interestingly, these calorie-burn figures compared to the hour's treadmill run (the runners covered about 9km in this time). The energy expenditure figures are high for all the test class types and demonstrate the significant calorie expenditure that boxing-based workouts can produce. Moreover, these boxing workouts are of a predominantly anaerobic nature and will require greater all over body power compared to treadmill running. This confirms

that these workouts are an effective way of developing general fitness, power and local muscular endurance under conditions of anaerobic fatigue.

If you find doing circuits difficult on your own, then a boxing circuit training class will not only get you motivated, but develop high levels of anaerobic and aerobic fitness, burn large numbers of calories and strengthen your body in ways that can benefit your running.

## Indoor rowing and running

Rowing uses nearly all the muscles in the body. It has a greater upper body requirement compared to running, with the shoulders and back in particular receiving a great workout, as well as the legs. The power for the rowing stroke, however, comes from the legs and is finished by the upper body (not as many people think from the arms). Good rowing technique is therefore crucial and you should spend time mastering it, before seriously using a machine as an adjunct to your run training (see panel on page 186).

### Benefits of rowing for runners as a cross-training option
- Rowing can maintain $VO_2$max.
- Rowing can develop all-over muscular strength, because of its greater upper body strength requirement.
- The rowing action is actually close to the running one (it requires a powerful leg action and extension of the ankles, hips and knees and the arm pull and uses the shoulders and upper back muscles in a not too dissimilar way to running (albeit all bilaterally as opposed to unilaterally).

### Suggestions for maximising the running cross-training benefits of rowing
*Add indoor rowing to your "base" building*
Middle, long and ultra-distance runners need to spend large amounts of their training developing a base of aerobic fitness. Exercise physiologists indicate that these athletes should do this at around 80 per cent of

### The Concept2 Rower
The most common rowing machine found in gyms up and down the country is the Concept2. These use air resistance produced through a fan mechanism that has a damper for adjustment. This should not be treated in the same way as a selector pin on a weights stack on a piece of fixed weight equipment, i.e. as a means to increase the intensity of your workout (although this can be an option for specific workouts, which are beyond the scope of this book). Rather, the setting should be utilised to establish your most efficient stroke. Most elite-level rowers will use a damper setting of 4/5.

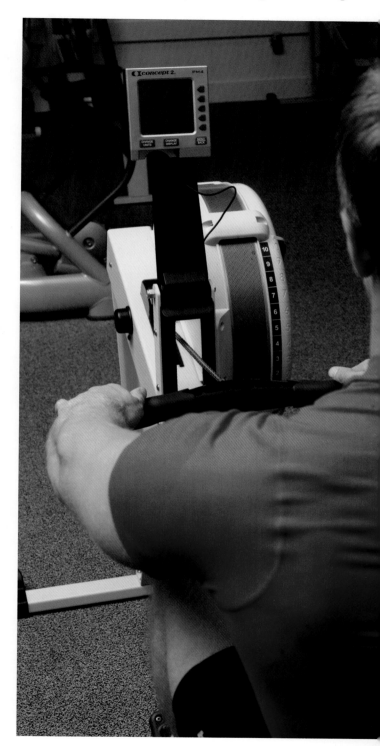

## Rowing/running ratio

A multiple of 0.75–1 should be used in favour of rowing – so the equivalent to a 30 minute run on a rower would be a 22.30 minute one, providing the same intensity was maintained (as measured by percentage of heart rate max, for example). It's important, as noted previously, that runners looking to use indoor rowing as relevant cross-training should learn to row technically correctly, as this will ensure optimal transference of rowing fitness into running fitness.

their maximum heart rate and that about 80 per cent of training should be completed in this zone. This will result in increased heart and lung efficiency, slow twitch (and fast twitch) muscle fibre oxygen processing ability and the ability to use more fat as a fuel source. Indoor rowing will benefit the middle, long and ultra-distance runner by contributing to the development and maintenance of a significant aerobic base, with a much-reduced risk of overuse injury (which we saw was one of the benefits of cycling). The following is a good example of an indoor rowing workout for aerobic endurance.

Work up from 2 x 5000m at 18–20 strokes per minute (SPM) at up to to 80 per cent MHR to 2 x 6000m to 3 x 5000m and finally 3 x 6000m at the same rate. Take 90 seconds' rest between each interval. Gradually periodise or build up these sessions over a 4-week period.

### Use the indoor rower to develop anaerobic fitness

Indoor rowing, as anyone who has attempted a 2k race (the Olympic distance) will know, can tax your energy systems like nothing else, well, except perhaps a 400m run or a 1500m race (the latter of which has similar aerobic/anaerobic requirements to the 2k rowing distance)!

If you race distances in particular between 800m and 5000m, then anaerobic conditioning is a must. You will

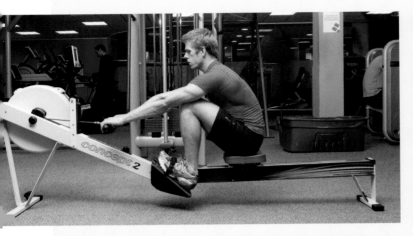

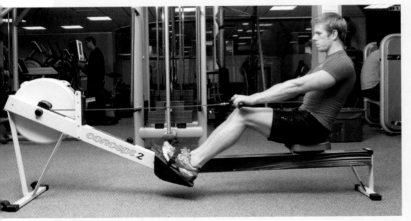

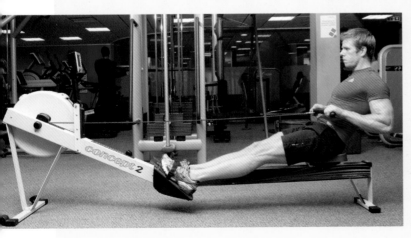

## Rowing technique

Machines do vary between manufacturers in terms of their set-up, so if you are in doubt, speak to a gym instructor or personal trainer on how to use a particular model. Having said that, rowing technique should be identical irrespective of the manufacturer.

### Starting position
Take hold of the oar with an over-grasp, shoulder-width grip. Bend your knees to 90 degrees and have your heels off the bottom of the foot rests. Your trunk should be inclined and your arms fully extended. The foot rest straps should be adjusted to allow your ankle to flex and extend as it pivots.

### The drive
Push your heels down into the foot rests and extend your legs to drive your body back down the slide. Resist the temptation to pull with your arms – instead keep them relaxed and extended and let your legs do the work. Try to keep the chain and the oar near parallel to the slide. When the oar passes your knees, then pull on it with your arms as you pivot back over your hips. Finish the stroke with your elbows behind your back and the oar close to your lower chest. Extend your arms to "push" the oar away and then flex your knees to return down the slide, into what's known as the "catch", ready for the next stroke. Keep your head up throughout and if the design of the rowing machine allows, position the monitor at head height. As with running the more relaxed you are the more efficient your technique will be.

need to develop your energy systems so they can tolerate significant lactate/lactic acid build-up whilst running at high speeds. Rowing can generate similar levels of anaerobic fatigue, and it will condition the mind as well as the muscles to tolerate this. Below are a selection of sample indoor rowing workouts designed to improve anaerobic capacity.

1  6 x 90 seconds at 95 per cent rowing intensity, 28–34SPM with 2 minutes gentle rowing recovery between efforts (at the end of each effort your heart rate should be around 90 per cent of MHR)
2  60 seconds
   90 seconds
   120 seconds
   90 seconds
   60 seconds
   Each effort should be completed at 90 per cent rowing intensity with an average heart rate of 80–85 per cent MHR, using 24–28 SPM and 60 seconds' slow rowing recovery between efforts.
3  15 minute increasing effort row
   Divide the 15 minutes into 3-minute sections. Begin at 2:05/500m pace and then increase your pace by 5 seconds/500m every 3 minutes, increasing stroke rate to handle the greater speeds as required.

   Target 3-minute splits would therefore be:
   2:05/500m pace at 20–22 SPM
   2:00/500m at 22 SPM
   1:55/500m at 24 SPM
   1:50/500m at 26 SPM
   1:45/500m at 28 SPM

Note: To successfully complete these sessions you will need to develop sufficient "understanding" of pace judgment on the indoor rower, as you would on the track or road when running. As you get more and more experienced, this will help you to develop your judgement.

## Maximum heart rate (MHR), running and rowing

Your maximum heart rate (MHR) will vary between modes of exercise, but it will invariably be higher for running, primarily due to the impact forces involved. You should expect your rowing heart rate maximum to be around 10 beats lower compared to your running one. It's therefore important to know your MHR for both activities (and any other cross-training CV methods you might incorporate into your training programme) to work within complimentary heart rate training zones.

### How to discover your rowing MHR
You will need a heart rate monitor. After a suitable warm-up, begin rowing at a moderate to hard pace for 2 minutes, then increase your pace on a controlled basis for subsequent 2-minute periods. After four intervals you should be approaching your MHR. Continue to row until you cannot push yourself any further and record your heart rate – this will be your rowing-specific MHR (you can perform this test for other CV methods).

Do not perform the test when you are tired, or have little specific rowing familiarity.

## References
1  *Sports Medicine*, 1994;18(5):330-9
2  *Journal of Strength & Conditioning Research*, 2003;17(2):319-23
3  Noakes T (2003), *The Lore of Running*, 4th edn, Human Kinetics:298
4  *Medicine and Science in Sports and Exercise*, 1997 Dec; 29(12):1653-6

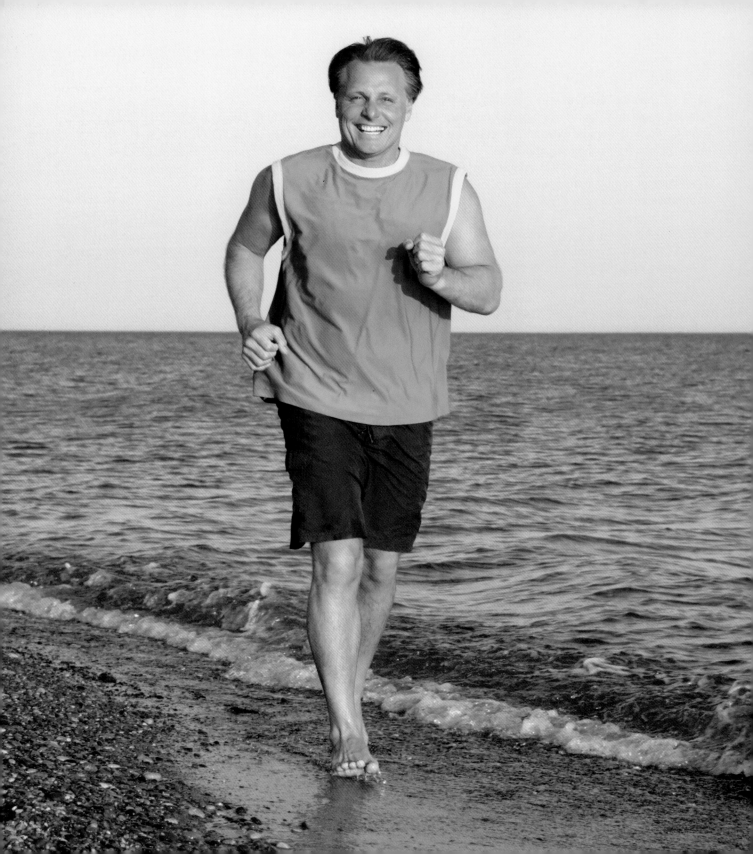

# 11
# strength training for the older runner

Running can be enjoyed at any age. There are those that run for a lifetime, those that start and stop and those that come to it in their middle and later years. In this chapter we will take a look at how to run "stronger for longer" with age. Tips, information and strategies are provided that are designed not only to keep you running strong, but also to combat the ageing process. It'll become apparent that running and exercise are very much the elixir of life!

"Master" runners officially start competing at the age of 35 and there are numerous races on the road and track at home and abroad, usually in five-year age bands for anyone above this age, up to 90 and even beyond (for more information, go to the British Masters Athletic Federation Website at www.bmaf.org.uk).

## Why does running speed decline with age?

A number of factors explain why we slow with age, however, particularly between the ages of 30 and 60, this decline need not be that great. Let's take a look at the negative factors first.

## Technique – stride length and stride frequency

Some of the major factors that result in a decrease in running speed relate to stride length. Researchers from Finland measured the performances of 70 finalists (males 40–88 years, females 35–87 years) at the European Veterans Athletics Championships in the year 2000 over the 100m sprint. The researchers measured, for example, velocity, stride length, stride rate, ground contact time and flight time, during the acceleration, maximum speed and deceleration phases of the sprint.[1]

Not surprisingly the researchers observed a general decline in sprint performance with age, which was particularly marked for the 65–70 year olds. Across the age groups, speed declined on average by 5–6 per cent per decade in men and 5–7 per cent per decade in women. Key to this decline was a growing reduction in stride length, which of course resulted in an increase in ground contact time, although the stride rate remained largely unaffected (apart from in the oldest age groups). So, what the researchers found is that the ageing runner will gradually spend more time propelling himself forwards, whilst travelling a shorter distance on each stride. Not great news. The most positive outcome, i.e. the retention of stride rate, can partly be explained by the fact that neural factors – particularly nerve conductivity – decline less significantly with age compared to other physiological determinants of speed production. Essentially, this means that older runners can still command their limbs to move at relatively high speeds, albeit unfortunately with much reduced power output and technical efficiency (especially if nothing is done to specifically condition against this, by way of relevant training and conditioning).

Further research into why runners slow with age corroborates the Finnish study. An American team compared 35–39-year-old runners with 90 year olds and noted a 40 per cent difference in stride length between the two age groups.[2] Specifically, the average stride length (for a two-stride cycle, i.e. the left and then the right leg) declined from 4.72m per stride (2.36m per step) to 2.84m per stride (just 1.42m per step). What this means is that a 90 year old needs to take nearly twice as many steps in the 100m compared to a 35 year old! The US researchers also confirmed the Finnish finding that stride frequency does not decline significantly with age.

## Declining muscle mass

With age, muscles shrink, a situation that is made worse for running by the fact that fast twitch fibres are lost in particular, which means less speed and power capability. In comparison, slow twitch fibres have greater longevity. In terms of fibre decline, the biceps muscle of a newborn baby has around 500,000 muscles fibres, while an 80 year old has 300,000. This loss of muscle fibre results in a greatly reduced capacity to express speed, strength and power. It is therefore important for the middle aged and older runner to continue to weight train (or start to do so, if they have not before). Doing plyometric exercises can also reduce the reduction in speed and power that comes with ageing (see page 193 for selected workouts).

Performing sprint drills will do much to keep your running technique as intact as it can be as you age (see chapter 3). These exercises will also strengthen your running muscles, ligaments and tendons and make

## Supplement with creatine

The supplement creatine can offer the middle and older aged runner (and anaerobic sprinter in the same age groups), who resistance trains and performs other anaerobic workouts in particular, added benefits in terms of maintaining muscle mass. Creatine allows for the completion of more repetitions and more forceful repetitions. It is a natural substance found in meat and fish and is a body chemical involved in anaerobic energy production. It can't be consumed in sufficient quantities to derive its optimum benefits so, by putting more of it in your system, specifically your muscles, you can train longer and stronger and with less fade when it comes to resistance training and other anaerobic training. This combined with a relevant resistance training programme can help to counter age-related muscles mass loss and improve running speed.

**Note:** Very little research, if any, indicates that creatine can be of assistance to aerobic training. Creatine requires a loading period and then a maintenance dose. Follow the manufacturer's instructions. Creatine is sold as a separate supplement and is also packaged with others to provide additional benefits. If you suffer from kidney problems in particular, you should seek advice before supplementing with creatine.

them more injury resilient, which will contribute towards your running longevity.

## Less growth hormone and testosterone are produced

With less of these androgens (growth hormone and testosterone), muscles lose their ability to gain in strength and size as a result of training and recovery from training and competition takes longer. The general decline in these hormones also contributes to the increased rate of ageing.

## Energy supply slows down

The supply of important energy producing body chemicals also declines with age, for example, creatine phosphate (CP). CP is the premium ingredient in muscles for short bursts of anaerobic physical activity, lasting 6–10 seconds. Less CP means that the ability to tackle high-intensity interval workouts declines with age. However, supplementing with creatine can boost its levels (see box above), as can the regular performance of short/high intensity weights, circuits and anaerobic CV interval training workouts.

An example running workout would involve 6–10 x 6om flat out sprints with a walk back recovery or 6 x 30 second sprints, performed at 90 per cent effort, with a 3-minute recovery between runs.

## Flexibility declines

Flexibility declines with age as soft tissue (muscles, ligaments and tendons) harden and joints stiffen. It is important to arrest this decline, not only for running performance, but also for future quality of life and mobility. Unless something is done, the loss can be as much as 30 per cent by the age of 70.

## Aerobic capacity reduces

The ability of the heart and lungs to produce energy declines from age 20, so much so that a 65 year old may possess only 65 per cent of his or her peak aerobic capacity. However, of all the markers of endurance running performance, aerobic capacity is the one that

## Further supplements

There are a number of supplements that can help manage joint deterioration, such as chondroitin and glucosamine sulphate. These supplements can reduce joint narrowing. They need to be constantly taken as their effects are preventative and long term. Research also indicates that they can reduce joint pain over time. It's certainly worth experimenting with them. As with creatine, seek medical advice before commencing any supplement routine.

declines the least between the ages of 30 and 60 and beyond if a concerted effort is made to maintain it.

## The effects of previous training

Many master runners may have been training for decades and, while this training will have provided numerous positive health and sporting benefits, the constant loading on their joints may also have had created some negative effects, for example, osteoarthritis. A great deal of research has shown that there is a correlation between years of participation in sport and osteoarthritis.

Osteoarthritis is a degenerative condition of the joints which become painfully inflamed. If there is joint degeneration without pain, the condition is known as osteoarthrosis. With both conditions, joint cartilage deteriorates. Cartilage is a smooth substance that covers bone endings, allowing them to glide over each other with minimal friction. Cartilage also cushions force when it is transmitted through joints. It serves a very similar function to the oil in your car engine, except that you can't top it up!

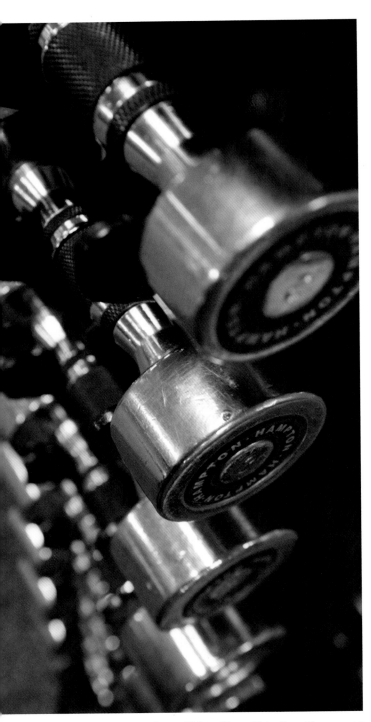

**Training with weights will be of benefit to the older runner**

# How to train to become a stronger older runner

## Weight train

We looked at weight training in detail in chapter 8. It's role is, if anything, even more important for older runners than it is for younger ones in terms of maintaining running ability and lean body mass. It'll also have a potentially profound effect on the general quality of later life.

As we discovered, muscle mass declines with age and this affects fast twitch fibre more significantly than slow twitch muscle fibre. However, regardless of age you can still do a lot to counteract this decline. Numerous research studies indicate that the body will respond to weight training irrespective of age. Studies involving 90 year olds have seen them double their leg strength after an appropriate training programme. Such has been the improvement in some of the participant's cases that they have been able to throw away their walking aids and walk unassisted. Don't put off weight training because you thinks it's too late – it's not.

### Weight train to boost growth hormone (GH) and testosterone

Weight training will also promote a positive hormonal response, which will create numerous positive outcomes for the master speed athlete.

As we have seen, growth hormone (GH) production declines with age. GH is involved in numerous anabolic functions relating to cell proliferation and division throughout the body, i.e. it stimulates the growth of bone, cartilage and muscle and can have positive effects on your lean muscle-to-fat ratio. In short, it can help build and maintain a leaner, stronger more powerful and less injury prone body.

Research suggests that high volume, moderate-to-high-intensity weight training, using relatively short rest intervals involving large amounts of muscle mass (i.e. using multi-joint, compound exercises, such as squats and lunges), produces the greatest rises in GH levels. This offers much for the older runner. This is because by boosting GH release, powerful and dynamic weight

## Weight training workouts designed to boost hormone levels and combat the ageing process

- 3 x 8 fast repetitions at 75% per cent 1RM, with incomplete recovery using compound (multi-joint) exercises, such as leg presses and squats.
- 3–5 x 4–6 fast repetitions at 80 per cent 1RM, with complete recovery (lifts as above).

*Fast* means powerful – movements which emphasise speed of movement. Try lifting and lowering to a 1:1 count. However, be sure to maintain control throughout the lift to avoid injury.

*Incomplete recovery* means that recovery between sets and exercises should be slightly less than needed – this will increase the intensity of the workout and the associated androgen response.

Note: Fast interval training workouts performed on a rowing machine or on a cycle as well as by running/ sprinting, will also create a very positive anabolic hormonal response (see page 192 for more information on the hormonal benefits of weight training).

training workouts can enhance muscle growth (or at least maintenance). This will reduce age-related decline and enable more powerful movements to be produced, which will be of benefit to running and everyday mobility, not to mention a possible slower age-related decline in general physical appearance.

Testosterone is an equally powerful anabolic hormone, produced by the testes in men and the ovaries in women. Research shows that, like GH, testosterone production is also stimulated by exercise. This is important, since the primary role of testosterone is to augment the release of GH.

Researchers from Finland specifically considered testosterone and GH response to weight training in master athletes. The survey's participants – 42 middle-aged and elderly men and women – completed six months of heavy resistance training. The researchers discovered that training led to significant rises in testosterone levels in both male groups, but not in the female groups. GH levels, however, increased in all groups, except the oldest women.

In terms of overall training response, 1RM (the maximum amount they could lift once) increased in the middle-aged men (average age 42) by 27 per cent; in the elderly men (average 72) by 16 per cent; in the

middle-aged women (average 39) by 28 per cent and in the elderly women (average 67) by 24 per cent.[3]

## Plyometric training and the older runner

Plyometric training is a great way to develop greater power and speed. Its performance relies on fast twitch muscle fibre, whose loss has been identified as a reason for older runners slowing with age. Weight training is important in terms of maintaining fast twitch muscle fibre and so is plyometric training. Older runners may argue that the stresses these exercises place on their body make them unsuitable, and it is true that the impact from plyometrics can be many times that of the performer's body weight (three plus times body weight), however, the same is also true of running.

On page 168, various plyometric exercises were ranked by intensity (the load they placed on the body, not their effectiveness). The lower intensity plyometric exercises would make for a highly suitable choice for inclusion in an age-combating resistance training plan. Such exercise would include those using a low trajectory, such as those performed over lines on the ground. Here are some examples:

# Ex 11.1 Double footed lateral line jump

**Intensity**
Low-medium

**How to perform**
Stand sideways onto a line and jump laterally over it, to land on your forefeet. Control the landing, i.e. don't fall across the line and power back to the start position. Repeat. The lateral movement will require ankle, calf strength and glute medius strength (the outer hip muscles) in particular, to brace against the lateral movements involved (if you have not trained these muscles regularly and dynamically, then progress carefully – see chapter 9 for core exercises that will strengthen the glute medius and chapter 1 for exercises designed to develop improved lower limb condition and awareness).

**Progression**
Perform on one leg at a time.

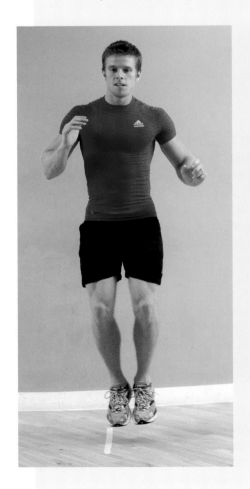
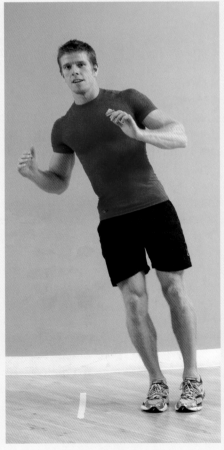
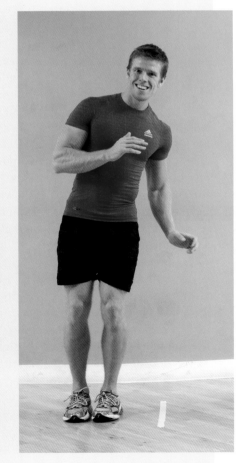

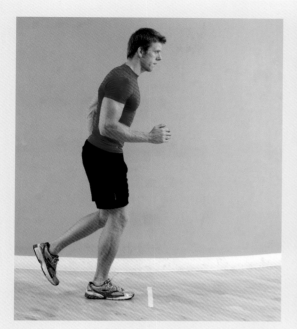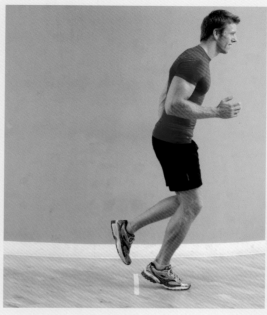

## Ex 11.2 Single leg lateral – side-to-side jumps

**Intensity**
Medium

**How to perform**
Stand side onto the line on one foot, having tucked the heel of the other up towards your bottom. Jump over the line, land on your forefoot and push back to hop back to where you started from. As exercise 11.1, look straight ahead and react as quickly as you can. Co-ordinate your arms with your legs.

### Progress plyometrics slowly
Always progress plyometric training gradually and emphasise quality of performance over quantity. 2 x 6–8 reps of two of the above exercises (or others selected) would be a sensible starting point for someone new to these exercises. Including them in your warm-up is a good option (see chapter 4).

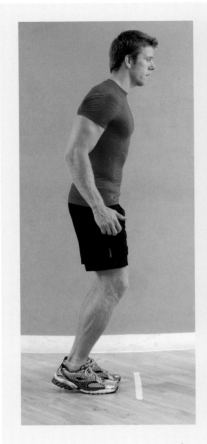
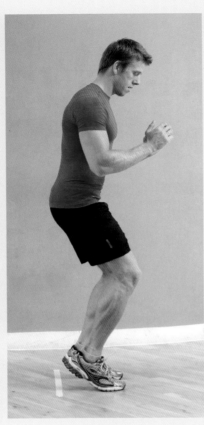

## Ex 11.3 Line bounce

**Intensity**
Medium

**How to perform**
Start with feet shoulder-width apart, close to and facing a line on an athletics track, sports hall floor or similar. With only a slight knee bend, jump over the line to land on your forefeet using a low trajectory. On landing, push back from your forefeet to jump back over the line to where you started. Land and repeat and develop a fast dynamic rhythm. Use your arms to aid balance and power. Try to look straight ahead and react as quickly as you can.

## Pre-conditioning is crucial for the older runner

Following a pre-conditioning routine as an older runner is very important (see chapter 1). The specific exercises will shore up and strengthen your body and combat many of the common injuries that can prevent running into middle and older age. The eccentric calf lowering exercise (see page 8) is a particularly useful exercise in this respect, as it can reduce Achilles tendon problems. Cross-training (see chapter 10) is also a vital weapon in the older runner's training armory, as is (hopefully!) a wise-head on old shoulders.

When it comes to running into old age in particular, a less-is-more approach is by far the best one to follow.

Enjoy your running, don't force yourself to complete greater and greater mileage and perform other training and fitness activities that will keep you running and generally as fit and healthy as you can be.

## References

1   *British Journal of Sports Med v.40(7); Jul 2006*
2   *Journal of Applied Biomechanics*, 1993(9):15-26
3   Hakkinen and team J Gerontol, *A Biol Sci Med Sci*, 2000 Feb;55(2):B95–105

# index